Creativity and Psychoanalytic Psychotherapy at Times of War, Exile, and Trauma

Creativity and Psychoanalytic Psychotherapy at Times of War, Exile, and Trauma draws upon decades of clinical experience to illuminate the unique challenges and profound insights that emerge when practising psychoanalytic psychotherapy within a multifaceted social terrain.

With reference to clinical case material and theoretical insight, Alfandary offers readers unprecedented access to therapeutic work conducted in Israel amid ongoing cultural tensions, military conflicts, and intergenerational trauma. Drawing from Winnicott, Bion, Klein, and Freud, the author explores how exile, trauma, and war fracture both individual identity and the social fabric, and how these ruptures can also spark unexpected creativity and growth. The book also covers a range of themes, including immigration, cross-cultural work, Holocaust memory, military trauma, and antisemitism, revealing how psychoanalytic practice adapts and responds to Israel's distinctive social pressures while offering universal insights into human resilience, trauma recovery, and the therapeutic relationship.

Creativity and Psychoanalytic Psychotherapy at Times of War, Exile, and Trauma will be of great interest to psychoanalytic psychotherapists, social workers, and psychologists. It will also be relevant for academics and scholars of Holocaust and trauma studies, literary studies, and interdisciplinary researchers.

Rony Alfandary, Ph.D., is a clinical social worker and senior lecturer at the School of Social Work at the University of Haifa, Israel. He served as Director of the Post-Graduate Programme in Psychoanalytic Psychotherapy at Bar-Ilan University until 2022. He is the author of twelve books, including prose and poetry.

"Rony Alfandary, whose previous book powerfully traced the legacy of his own family's experiences during Nazi times, has written another open and compelling text, this time developing his ideas on the practice of psychoanalytic psychotherapy in Israel. With the aid of semi-fictionalised clinical 'cases' along with literary and social analysis, Alfandary explores how psychoanalytic practice can articulate the fraught context of one of the most trauma-saturated communities in the world. The book raises issues around trauma, inheritance, antisemitism and war and will be of value to all who are interested in the practice and politics of psychoanalysis."

Stephen Frosh, *Emeritus Professor, Birkbeck, University of London*

"Alfandary's book, drawing on decades of experience in the shadow of war, offers an original and illuminating interweaving of two healing threads, ethics and creativity, forming a generous, lucid, and deeply human guide to psychotherapy, trauma, and recovery. Through Alfandary's remarkable gift for storytelling, it stands as a compassionate testimony to the enduring human capacity for repair and to its hard-won restoration along the psychotherapeutic path in times of trauma and exile."

Prof. Roth Merav, Ph.D., *training psychoanalyst and cultural researcher, University of Haifa, International Sigourney award winner, 2024*

"Rony Alfandary, a prominent figure in Israel's mental health field, combines in this powerful book his insights regarding attributes of Israeli society – the shadow of the Holocaust, experiences of migration, the traumatic impact of wars and terrorism, political struggles between democratic and authoritarian forces – with his thinking about the universal aspects of psychoanalytic psychotherapy and of clinical social work. His emphasis on the creative significance of psychotherapy is expressed in unique case studies and in explorations of the potential contribution of literature and music."

Emanuel Berman, Ph.D., *Israel Psychoanalytic Society*

Creativity and Psychoanalytic Psychotherapy at Times of War, Exile, and Trauma

Rony Alfandary

Routledge
Taylor & Francis Group
LONDON AND NEW YORK

Designed cover image: © Edith Reisner Alfandary, A Place on the Horizon

First published 2026
by Routledge
4 Park Square, Milton Park, Abingdon, Oxon OX14 4RN

and by Routledge
605 Third Avenue, New York, NY 10158

Routledge is an imprint of the Taylor & Francis Group, an informa business

British Library Cataloguing-in-Publication Data
A catalogue record for this book is available from the British Library

ISBN: 978-1-041-16178-3 (hbk)
ISBN: 978-1-041-16177-6 (pbk)
ISBN: 978-1-003-68316-2 (ebk)

DOI: 10.4324/9781003683162

Typeset in Times New Roman
by Taylor & Francis Books

Contents

Introduction

On 13th August, 1937, as Nazi forces gathered at the borders of Austria, Sigmund Freud (1856–1939) wrote a letter to his friend and patron Marie Bonaparte (1882–1962). In it, he reflected on a question that many have asked in times of despair: the meaning of life itself.

> *The moment a man questions the meaning and value of life, he is sick, since objectively neither has any existence; by asking this question one is merely admitting to a store of unsatisfied libido to which something else must have happened, a kind of fermentation leading to sadness and depression.*
>
> (Freud, 1960, p. 436)

These words carry the weight of a man who had dedicated his career to understanding suffering and was now facing his own mortality. For Freud, the very act of questioning existence was not philosophy but a signal of unrest, a symptom of the human condition when it confronts forces beyond comprehension.

This book is based upon a similar place of questioning, though almost a century later, in a different part of the world. It was written in Israel, during a time marked by the COVID-19 pandemic, massive public protests, and the devastation of 7th October, 2023, and the ensuing war. These events prompted me, as a clinical social worker and psychoanalytic psychotherapist, to ask how therapy can respond to collective trauma while staying true to the intimate work of healing individual lives.

The title, *Creativity and Psychoanalytic Psychotherapy at Times of War, Exile, and Trauma*, captures the central themes. *War* destroys any sense of safety. *Exile* robs people of belonging. *Trauma* fragments continuity of self and history. Yet, from these very ruptures, profound possibilities for creativity and growth can emerge. The book explores these possibilities through case studies, theory, literature, and personal reflection.

The Wounded Healer

Carl Jung (1875–1961) described therapists as *wounded healers*, borrowing from the Greek myth of Chiron, a healer who could not heal his own wound. To become a psychotherapist, one must first have faced pain in one's own life. In Israel, this idea is more than symbolic. Therapists and clients live in the same conditions of constant uncertainty, war, and social unrest. These raise pressing questions: How can one remain neutral when one's own community is under attack? How can one treat trauma while living in a society founded by exiles and still producing new displacements?

These are not abstract questions. They have shaped my 34 years of clinical practice. The fictionalized cases in this book are drawn from those experiences. Sue, a Filipina caregiver, grieves a miscarriage while far from home. Vered, an Israeli paratrooper, carries not only her own trauma but also her grandmother's memories of the Holocaust. David, in exile, uses literature and film to navigate depression. Gil, a teenager, finds containment for his struggles in the music of Pink Floyd's *Wish You Were Here* and The Who's *Tommy*. These stories show how therapy must move between the intimate and the historical, between the private self and public crisis.

In this context, creativity is more than making art. It is the capacity to work with whatever materials life offers, however painful, and to find one's own voice in response. For both individuals and societies, creativity becomes a survival tool. When familiar structures collapse, through pandemic, war, or social upheaval, people must improvise new ways of making meaning. Protest, testimony, music, literature, and even the therapeutic relationship itself are creative acts that can transform suffering into something bearable and communicable.

The Architecture of Disruption

The chapters that follow are arranged around what might be called *an architecture of disruption*: the ways breakdowns in personal, social, and political life create openings for new forms of practice and understanding.

The first four chapters examine the ethical and methodological foundations of therapy in unstable conditions. How do we listen when trauma has shattered language itself? How do we write about clients in ways that protect both truth and dignity? What does it mean to begin therapy in the midst of ongoing crisis?

Chapters Five to Eight deal with clinical dilemmas where traditional boundaries fall short. In one case, Amanda's erotic transference turns into a defence against intimacy itself. In David's treatment, literature and film become a transitory space, an *analytic third*, that makes communication possible across displacement. Gil's identification with the deaf, dumb, and blind protagonist of *Tommy* shows how popular culture can help metabolize trauma when family fails to provide emotional containment.

The last three chapters widen the lens. Vered's panic attacks during reserve duty open up questions of intergenerational trauma and the ethics of bearing witness. Reflections on Aharon Appelfeld (1932–2018), Lawrence Durrell (1912–1990), and Freud reveal how displacement can bring both loss and creative possibility. The study of Israel's COVID-19 protests shows how societies under pressure swing between authoritarian and democratic impulses.

The book concludes with my own responses to 7th October, 2023, as both therapist and citizen. In that moment, neutrality became impossible. The work included providing trauma treatment, documenting testimonies, supporting IDF families, and maintaining dialogue across ethnic divides. Here, therapy was not a retreat from politics but a form of civic engagement.

Psychoanalysis as Creative Practice: The Return of the Repressed

A central argument runs throughout this book: psychoanalytic psychotherapy is not only treatment but also a creative practice that makes meaning out of suffering.

This perspective draws on the British School tradition, Donald Winnicott (1896–1971), Wilfred Bion (1897–1979), and Melanie Klein (1882–1960), while remaining rooted in Freud's drive theory and enriched by interdisciplinary and intersubjective approaches.

Therapy, in this view, begins not with interpretation but with listening, even to what cannot yet be spoken. In trauma and exile, meaning often exists only in silences, pauses, or fragmented gestures. The therapist's task is to create language that respects, rather than reduces, this complexity.

Bion's idea of *the container and contained* is central: the therapeutic relationship must provide a holding space for unbearable experiences, metabolizing them without being overwhelmed. Literature, music, and film are not just illustrations but part of this process, especially when words fail.

Psychological symptoms never exist in isolation. They are entangled with wider social, cultural, and historical forces. Effective therapy, therefore, must address both the inner world and the outer context that shapes it.

Across the cases, a pattern emerges that Freud described as *the return of the repressed*. Unprocessed trauma resurfaces in new forms. Vered's panic during military service echoes her grandmother's Holocaust terror. David's depression in exile resonates with generations of Jewish displacement. Gil's identification with a numb, damaged character mirrors his father's silence after war.

This pattern also appears on a collective scale. After 7th October, antisemitism surged globally, and Israel adopted some of the violence it was attacked by. Through Klein's concept of *projective identification*, this can be seen as societies under stress projecting unwanted parts of themselves onto others. Similarly, Israel's COVID-19 protests, understood through Mikhail Bakhtin's (1895–1973) notion of carnival, reveal how democratic dissent uses humour, inversion, and parody to challenge authority.

Such dynamics suggest that Freud's insights into individual psychology may apply even more powerfully to collective life. Concepts like *repetition compulsion, reaction formation*, and *the uncanny* illuminate both personal symptoms and social movements.

Beyond the Consulting Room: The Courage to Continue

This book does not claim political neutrality. I write as an Israeli Jewish clinical social worker in a time of crisis. I openly affirm democratic values, equal national and civil rights to all people in the Middle East, pluralism, non-violence, and the duty to bear witness. This reflects what Jessica Benjamin (b. 1946) calls *mutual recognition*.

Neutrality itself, I argue, can become a political stance when democracy is under threat. Drawing on Hannah Arendt's (1906–1975) distinction between *labour, work*, and *action*, I see therapeutic practice as extending beyond the clinic into civic engagement. This does not mean imposing politics on clients but recognizing that therapy is always entangled with the social and political fabric in which it takes place.

In moments of upheaval, the therapist's ability to hold curiosity, hope, and compassion becomes a form of social repair. The consulting room is not separate from the world; it is one of the places where democratic values, dialogue, respect, and recognition are either sustained or lost.

Throughout this book, literature serves as more than background. Freud's letters from exile, Albert Camus's (1913–1960) *The Plague*, Julio Cortázar's (1914–1984) vision of estrangement, Lawrence Durrell's prose, and Aharon Appelfeld's writings all provide models for how displacement and crisis can be transformed into meaning.

This reflects my conviction that psychoanalysis and literature share a task: turning raw, often chaotic experience into narrative. Both practices rely on what Paul Ricoeur (1913–2015) called *the hermeneutics of suspicion*, the sense that surface meanings hide deeper truths that require interpretation.

The Israeli context gives this method particular urgency. In a society founded by refugees, shaped by conflict, and composed of immigrants alongside indigenous Palestinians, the line between personal and collective memory is always unstable. Identity itself becomes a creative, ongoing project.

This book was written in a time when professional, political, and personal frameworks felt increasingly insufficient. It does not promise easy solutions or universal techniques. Instead, it is an attempt to remain engaged with the hardest questions:

How do we create in the face of loss? How do we hope when despair seems overwhelming? How do we maintain dignity when forces beyond our control strip it away?

The Jewish tradition of *tikkun olam*, repairing the world, provides one guiding thread. Healing begins with the individual but must extend to the collective.

Lawrence Durrell once said he lived his life pretending; he improvised between cultures, neither fully Indian nor British. This improvisation, far from failure, may be the most truthful response to modern life. We are all displaced, piecing together homes from theory, art, politics, relationships, and memory.

The chapters in this book document such improvisations: in the consulting room, in supervision, in protests, and in responses to historical catastrophe. They testify that even in the darkest times humans retain the capacity to create meaning, sustain relationships, and act with compassion.

This persistence is not inevitable. It requires daily renewal, the courage to remain open to painful experience, and the will to continue creating.

Freud suggested to Marie Bonaparte that questioning life's meaning may be a sign of sickness. But it may also be the beginning of health, the recognition that meaning is not discovered but created. To live, love, and bear witness is itself the work of creating meaning.

This book is offered in that spirit, not as certainty but as continued questioning. Not as answers but as an invitation to keep engaging with the uncertainty that defines human existence.

A Note to Readers

I wrote this book primarily for professional communities in Israel and worldwide who work with people under stress. But I also hope it will interest anyone concerned with the human condition.

To make the reading flow more smoothly, I placed the bibliography at the very end, rather than using academic footnotes. While the book was written as a whole, each chapter is designed to stand on its own, so readers can approach it in parts.

The views expressed here are mine alone, but they were shaped by the shared experiences of my clients, peers, teachers, and students. I deeply thank all the good people at Routledge who have made this book possible.

I am grateful to my wife and two sons, whose continuing support provides me with the space necessary for writing. I dedicate this book to my family, my community, and to all human beings in the world with the hope that the world remains a place of love, safety, and inspiration.

A Note to Readers

Chapter 1

Listening to a Whisper

Psychoanalytic Social Work and the Ethics of Representing Inner Experience

Psychoanalytic literature is rich with reflections on the dark dimensions of the human mind – those territories where language loses its bearings. Acts of cruelty, self-destructive compulsions, sadism, and perversion are often conceptualized as expressions of early emotional damage, formed in primitive developmental stages where something essential went wrong. These phenomena are not merely pathological but echo deeper, often silent, catastrophes lodged at the foundations of the self.

Psychoanalytic psychotherapists are often confronted with such emotional states that defy articulation, sessions that evoke a sense of helplessness and disrupt their personal and professional sense of *agency*. In such moments, there is a tendency to retreat into rigid diagnostic categories, as if severe classifications might contain what resists understanding. Sigmund Freud poignantly addressed this dilemma in his 1937 essay *Analysis Terminable and Interminable*, where he reflected on the bedrock of personality and acknowledged that certain emotional conditions may lie beyond the conventional therapeutic reach.

Psychoanalytic psychotherapy is indeed neither the ultimate nor the exclusive path to understanding emotional disturbance or human behaviour. There remain actions and inner states that resist comprehension, elude symbolic description, evade clear solutions, and confront us with the limits of our profession.

In this opening chapter, I will outline my argument that it is nevertheless the task, and indeed the ethical responsibility, of the informed *psychoanalytic psychotherapist* to continuously strive towards giving clear verbal expression to all sensual, emotional, and cognitive experience, whether these are hidden, repressed, or silenced.

That is what we do when we practise psychoanalytic psychotherapy: we give expression to that which has eluded articulation, what has been denied exposure due to internal inhibitions, unresolved conflicts, emotional wounds, and external forces such as prohibition and stigma.

We must resist the temptation to hide behind the claim that certain mental phenomena are beyond words or description. This is not to suggest that we

DOI: 10.4324/9781003683162-1

possess absolute knowledge, but rather that we are committed to the relentless pursuit of understanding. Our task is to ground our work in clearly expressed and rational concepts, and not to mask our uncertainty with obscure or mystifying language.

The Relevance of Psychoanalytic Psychotherapy

In the following pages, I will explore the various theoretical concepts and contexts that have shaped my work as a clinical social worker practising psychoanalytic psychotherapy with children, adolescents, and adults over the past 34 years in Israel. I believe that my own personal experience, based upon my training in the UK and Israel, reflects the challenges faced by other therapists around the world, despite the obvious geographical and cultural differences.

The scope of this chapter, and the book, cannot do justice to the magnitude and depth of all the concepts I shall discuss. I have chosen to illuminate a theoretical path which I believe is a practical one and offers inspiration and perhaps even guidance to therapists at whatever stage of their career. The list of concepts I selected is by no means exhaustive, and I know that there are many more which are as important. My choice has been mainly guided by what concepts have helped me consistently to understand my practice and to continuously improve it. It is not a linear path at times, but I hope that an authentic, coherent, and useful theoretical path is being suggested.

It is important to emphasize from the outset that psychoanalytic psychotherapy is not confined to private clinics or mental health centres. Psychoanalytic social workers and other mental health professionals work in a wide range of settings, whether in residential facilities, welfare offices, correctional services, or elsewhere, and with diverse populations such as children, refugees, survivors of sexual abuse, or individuals from disadvantaged socioeconomic backgrounds (from this point onwards, I will use the term therapist to refer to the diverse groups of mental health professionals practising psychoanalytic psychotherapy, including social workers, psychologists, psychiatrists, art therapists, and clinical criminologists). They can all be inspired by the core concepts of psychoanalytic theory. These basic ideas, which I will explore in the following pages, address directly the question that guides my practice: *what is it that I do when I do what I do?*

The fundamental premise of this chapter, and indeed of the entire book, is that the various psychoanalytic theories developed since the early 20th century continue to offer both theoretical inspiration and practical guidance for all therapists.

In the following pages, I suggest a few conceptual elaborations which offer a wide framework for examining how we operate as therapists. Together, they constitute a possible response to the fundamental question I have posed: *what is it that I do when I do what I do*? The concepts and ideas introduced here will be developed and contextualized throughout the subsequent chapters, where I aim to demonstrate their practical applicability and clinical relevance through detailed fictional case studies and theoretical and cultural exploration.

I make no claim to originality in the way I present the framework, recognizing my profound debt to the many colleagues and teachers who have provided inspiration and knowledge throughout my professional development.

Our inner life is shaped by the constant flow through a matrix of three interweaving layers: sensations, emotions, and thoughts. Sensations are the raw data we receive from the body and the outside world, such as warmth, cold, pressure, or a racing heartbeat. They are the most immediate signals, telling us what is happening physically in any given moment. Emotions or feelings arise when the mind gives meaning to these sensations. For example, a tight chest and quick breath may be felt as anxiety, while a relaxed body may be experienced as calm or joy. Emotions are often more complex than sensations because they combine physical signals with personal history, memories, and unconscious associations.

Thoughts add yet another layer. They are the words and images we use to explain, justify, or question what we feel. A worried thought may intensify anxiety, while a hopeful thought may soften fear. Thoughts can shape emotions, and emotions can influence the kinds of thoughts that appear. For example, sadness may bring self-critical thoughts, while excitement may bring optimistic ones.

These three, sensations, emotions, and thoughts, are deeply interconnected. Becoming aware of their links allows us to pause, reflect, and respond more wisely, instead of being carried away by automatic reactions. All human experience involves body sensations, emotional recognition, and cognitive processing. The questions as to which of these layers affects us quicker is open to debate. It is tempting to think that we are initially motivated to action by our bodily sensations, but this is of course a tricky statement as we now know that the mind comes into existence alongside the body and therefore to claim precedence of one over the other can be disputed. Still, I suggest that it is a good-enough practical assumption and at least places the body firmly within our framework. Understanding this allows therapists to work with clients at whichever level of experience is most accessible or therapeutically relevant at any given moment.

As psychoanalytic psychotherapists, we are often in danger of forgetting the body and focusing too much on the mind. Noticing the body has been dealt with hesitation in the past, not least because it has led sometimes to ethical transgression. We must not go the other way and ignore the body.

We need to learn to listen to our sensations, our emotions, and thoughts with equal importance – bearing in mind that they all communicate with different speeds and frequencies – so that when we listen to a client who tells us of a scene of domestic violence, we need to be aware of how our body responds to such verbal messages and how our feelings adapt in the attempt to remain open towards experiences we find hard to digest and comprehend.

Freud postulated a fundamental split within every human mind between conscious awareness and unconscious motivation. While we prefer to believe we operate through reason and logic, we frequently find ourselves driven by forces outside our immediate awareness and control.

This conscious-unconscious distinction forms a central tenet of psychoanalytic theory. Early life experiences become embedded in the unconscious and shape our present and future patterns of behaviour, perception, and relationship. These experiential imprints form what we might call our *core sense of self*, often referred to in psychoanalytic terms as *fantasy*, the internalized world of memories, experiences, and relational patterns that continues to inform our consciousness throughout life.

Without developing awareness of these unconscious patterns, without recognizing that we often act according to internalized templates, object relations, and attachment styles, rather than responding rationally to present circumstances, we risk being controlled by forces stronger than our conscious will. The therapeutic goal is not to eliminate *fantasy* but to expand awareness of its influence and rely on its strength as a creative drive.

This awareness does not grant unlimited freedom and may even bring pain as we confront previously unconscious forbidden desires and repressed losses. However, it moves us towards living as more thoughtful, intentional beings. We spend our lives negotiating between this internalized *fantasy* world, which serves as both constraint and source of creativity, and the demands of present reality, striving to respond to current circumstances without being unduly influenced by echoes from the past.

Current psychoanalytic theories now rest upon an integrative synthesis between Freudian and post-Freudian models that conceptualizes the mind as composed of two intertwined structures: the intrapersonal (rooted in Freudian dual drive theory) and the interpersonal (developed through object relations theories).

The intrapersonal structure refers to the way our fundamental survival needs – and the extent to and manner in which they were met during early development – shape our internal psychological world and subsequent social relationships. In this framework, sexuality plays a central, though not exclusive, role in psychological development and motivation.

The interpersonal structure emphasizes that the specific qualities, behaviours, and emotional patterns of our early caregivers and the way they consistently responded to our needs become internalized unconsciously, forming relational templates that continue to inform our future behaviour, expectations, and relationship choices. These internalized *object relations* create an inner world populated by representations of significant others and their relationship dynamics.

These two conceptual frameworks are not contradictory but rather complementary, offering different lenses through which to understand human development. The primary distinction lies in the increasing significance that post-Freudian theorists have attributed to environmental factors in shaping individual development, moving beyond purely drive-based explanations to include the profound influence of relational experiences.

In many ways, the dynamic tension between these approaches reflects the broader nature versus nurture paradigm, with intrapersonal theories emphasizing innate drives and developmental stages, while interpersonal theories highlight the formative power of early relationships and environmental influences.

Practical Implications and Context

What are the practical implications of these theories?

If, as Freud proposed, we are inclined to repeat patterns established in early childhood, patterns of which we retain little conscious memory, then these tendencies inevitably resurface in our later relationships. Freud termed this dynamic *repetition compulsion*. Practising psychoanalytic psychotherapy, we offer a controlled container, some would call it a laboratory, where such repetitions and reenactments can emerge in real time through the phenomenon of *transference*. This makes therapy a rare opportunity to observe these patterns as they unfold, explore their origins, and experiment with new ways of relating.

In every meeting between two people, there exists some degree of repetition of past relational patterns. We are conditioned to experience the external world through what we already know of it. It is in a sense a comfort, being in a familiar world. This comfort is of course shattered when faced with stress and trauma as I will expand upon later. What distinguishes the therapeutic space from other areas in life where we meet this repetition is the therapist's recognition that this repetition constitutes the primary arena where personal conflicts are reenacted and can be examined.

According to this idea, the evolving relationship between therapist and client will meaningfully echo both the client's early developmental patterns and their current relationships with significant others. Often, determining who initiated what, whether the therapist's unconscious response to the client preceded the client's transference towards the therapist, or vice versa, proves nearly impossible. I therefore conceptualize *transference* as a mutual, bidirectional process. When we talk about transference, we encompass the totality of projections, identifications, and unconscious dynamics operating within the therapeutic dyad.

The therapeutic responsibility lies squarely with the therapist. They must regulate, understand, and interpret these transference processes in ways that make the unconscious content, reenactments, and relational patterns more accessible to the client's awareness. The exploration of what I call *the therapeutic triangle* – the client's current relationships, past patterns, and the therapeutic relationship – constitutes the core psychoanalytic therapeutic agenda.

Without romanticizing the therapeutic process or reducing its complexity, therapeutic action can be understood as operating through two primary mechanisms. The first is the establishment and maintenance of *the therapeutic setting*, discussed in detail in Chapter Three. The second consists of verbal interventions, including interpretation, in which sensory, emotional, and cognitive material is brought into resonance across all three vertices of the triangle, creating the conditions for a shared and collaborative exploration with the client.

The purpose of *interpretation* and the subsequent *working-through* of gained insights is to facilitate positive transformation of the debilitating *defence mechanisms* the client has developed. This process is inherently complex, far from inevitable, and often fails to achieve optimal results. Nevertheless, this represents the fundamental therapeutic aim: facilitating the client's development of more adaptive and fulfilling ways of being. The bulk of this book, Chapters Four to Eight, demonstrates specific instances of this therapeutic work in practice.

Psychotherapy always occurs within a specific cultural context that fundamentally shapes both the therapeutic process and its outcomes. It must be observed, acknowledged, and carefully considered both within the therapeutic relationship and in broader societal frameworks. This understanding cannot be relegated to background considerations but must remain central to therapeutic practice. There are several intersecting factors: the cultural backgrounds of both therapist and client, the social context in which therapy takes place, and the theoretical-ethical framework that guides the therapist's practice. The therapist must maintain acute awareness of both the sensitivity of these issues and their own relationship to them, including their positions of privilege, marginalization, or cultural difference relative to their clients.

These conceptual frameworks, while metaphorical and often difficult to verify scientifically, provide essential structure for clinical work. They allow therapists to maintain both confidence in their therapeutic approach and *a sense of agency* in navigating complex human dynamics. These theories transform therapeutic practice from reliance on intuition, goodwill, and chance into work grounded in systematic understanding of human psychological development and functioning.

This book is written from the perspective of a male Jewish clinical social worker practising psychoanalytic psychotherapy in Israel, trained in both the UK (where I was born) and Israel. These facts inform what I do. Over the past 34 years, since returning to Israel, I have worked as a social worker and psychotherapist with very diverse populations as I will hopefully demonstrate throughout this book.

Israel exists as a state founded through successive waves of Jewish immigration beginning in 1948, established in the aftermath of (though not exclusively due to) the Holocaust, while coexisting with the indigenous Palestinian population. Israel has been in an almost constant state of conflict, often violent, with its neighbouring countries. It also suffers deep inner conflicts between the different populations living within its borders. This complex historical and demographic reality makes cultural diversity and recognition crucial elements in understanding the therapeutic work presented throughout this book.

Several chapters throughout this book address different facets of this cultural dimension. The final two chapters directly address some of the specific historical circumstances during which this book was written, demonstrating how contemporary political and social realities inevitably permeate therapeutic space and theoretical understanding.

Being Fit for the Job

One of the most fundamental conditions that underlies the wide range of possible answers to the question I posed earlier (*what is it that I do when I do what I do*) is, quite simply, the presence of two people sharing the same space, whether physically or remotely, engaged in conversation. This may sound self-evident, and indeed it is, yet it bears repeating. Psychoanalytic theories can sometimes become so complex, abstract, or over-intellectualized that they obscure this essential, deeply human element of our work: we are having conversations, dialogues.

In this sense, psychotherapy is not altogether different from other conversations people have, even in times of distress. What distinguishes our practice is the theoretical framework we bring to bear. In this case it is the psychoanalytic concepts that help us interpret, understand, and give meaning to the content and process of these conversations. In this regard, psychotherapy can be seen as a sibling of the philosophical tradition known as *hermeneutics.*

Hermeneutics is the art of interpretation. Historically, it emerged from the interpretation of religious texts, aimed at uncovering hidden meanings within complex and often ambiguous writings. In modern times, thinkers such as Paul Ricoeur, Hans-Georg Gadamer (1900–2002) and Martin Heidegger (1889–1976) expanded its use to the interpretation of philosophical texts, cultural phenomena, and human experience more broadly.

Psychoanalytic psychotherapy shares with hermeneutics the basic belief that meaning is often concealed, embedded beneath the surface of words, actions, and silences, and that uncovering it requires a process of interpretation, whether through conversation or writing. In his view, psychoanalysis is a method of interpretation – *hermeneutics* of *suspicion* – that examines texts, actions, or social phenomena for hidden structures and unconscious motives. Drawing on Freud, Karl Marx (1818–1883), and Friedrich Nietzsche (1844–1900), Ricoeur suggests that the apparent meaning of words or actions often hides deeper mental and social forces. In psychoanalytic terms, what appears on the surface is like a symptom: it signals underlying conflicts, desires, or repressed content. For Freud, human behaviour is shaped by unconscious drives and repressed wishes. Marx adds a structural dimension, showing how economic and class forces shape consciousness, while Nietzsche highlights the role of hidden moral and psychological pressures. Ricoeur combines these perspectives to argue that interpretation must go beyond manifest content to uncover latent meanings.

In clinical or textual analysis, the hermeneutics of suspicion functions like a psychoanalytic reading: it seeks to reveal what is repressed, denied, or disavowed. Yet Ricoeur emphasizes that *suspicion* alone is not enough; interpretation should also move towards understanding – acknowledging the relationship between repression and recovery. By attending to the unconscious layer and latent content, his approach exposes the mental and social mechanisms that shape human thought, behaviour, and cultural expression.

Such an investigation of language and writing has been central to my development as a writer and psychotherapist. All the chapters in this book demonstrate this preoccupation. I regard literature and psychoanalysis as sibling disciplines, each grappling with the fundamental questions of human existence, and each offering bold, imaginative attempts to understand the inner life, whether through the intimacy of the therapy room or the solitude of reading.

To embark upon the dialogue that psychotherapy entails, and to give it the best possible chance of succeeding in its aims, namely alleviating human suffering and discovering meaning where pain resides, a safe and secure space must first be established, *a home*. Regardless of the physical locality in which this dialogue takes place, be it a welfare office, clinic, probation service, residential institution, community centre, children's home, or youth facility, there are both symbolic and concrete factors that must be considered.

The physical setting requires a room situated in a quiet environment, where the door can be closed and external distractions, such as loud noises or nearby traffic, are minimized. The space should offer comfortable seating, good lighting, and be accessible to all, ensuring physical ease and inclusiveness. More than just a room, this space becomes a kind of home for the therapeutic pair, home in the deeper, symbolic sense: a place where one feels seen, known, and understood, and to which one can return, even when it feels difficult to remain.

The symbolic elements essential to therapeutic practice resist easy categorization, constituting *the art of listening*, a concept explored in depth throughout this work. The capacity to listen is perhaps a natural human trait, and we may assume we can take it for granted. I suggest that this is not the case.

For the therapist to be able to listen, rather than just wait out the client's speech so that they can say what's on their mind, special care needs to be taken. Listening psychoanalytically require training and practice. Even though we all know how to hear what other people say, often we do not listen well enough to the myriad forms of communications that are delivered, consciously and unconsciously.

While it may seem self-evident, the therapist's fundamental fitness for this demanding role cannot be overstated. We cannot listen to someone else's story as therapists unless we are taking good-enough care of ourselves. We must work at having our own stories heard so that they do not impose themselves upon the client. As mentioned in the Introduction, therapists mostly choose this profession because of having had relevant personal experience. Such an experience must be explored during the initial training and later so that we know how to distinguish our own issues from those of the clients. As referred to throughout the book, repetition of past experiences is one of the main practices that occurs in therapy and therefore requires firm and sound self-knowledge to not burden the client with personal unresolved issues. In plain words, all therapists must be in supervision and personal therapy during the various stages of their career.

On Becoming an Ambivalent Adult

Traditionally, a distinction is being made between *transference*, i.e. what the client unconsciously projects onto the therapist, and *countertransference*, i.e. what the therapist projects onto the client. Though this distinction is valid and important, I suggest viewing the whole phenomena as one. *Transference* cannot exist without *countertransference* and vice versa. Therefore, throughout this book I will refer to the concept of *transference* as containing both.

As demonstrated in Chapters Three to Eight, the transference paradigm pervades every therapeutic session. This demands that therapists possess the capacity for profound self-examination, continuously monitoring their sensual, emotional, and cognitive processes to detect traces of repetition compulsion, projected unresolved conflicts, and other fundamental dynamics inherent in therapeutic relationships.

Transference is a core element in therapy but needs to be viewed as inherently fluid. Throughout therapeutic work, it consistently serves as a repository for unconscious material: clients project onto their therapists unresolved emotional patterns, conflicts, and relationship dynamics from their past. However, the specific manifestations of these projections are far from uniform or predictable.

The flexibility of transference becomes particularly evident when examining how the therapist's personal attributes shape what clients project onto them. Age is one example. When a client in their twenties meets with a therapist in their thirties, the unconscious material that emerges will likely differ significantly from what surfaces with a therapist in their sixties. The younger therapist might evoke projections related to sibling dynamics, peer relationships, or perhaps an idealized parent figure. As an example, the younger therapist might be seen as a sibling figure by a client of the same age, potentially triggering issues around envy, competition, and sexuality that differ markedly from the kind of projections triggered by an older therapist, which may have more to do with authority and parenthood.

Conversely, an older therapist naturally invites different unconscious projections. They may more readily become the recipient of parental transferences, embodying authority, wisdom, mortality, or disappointment in ways that reflect the client's early caregiver relationships. The male therapist might unconsciously represent different aspects of fatherhood, from protective authority to distant unavailability, depending partly on their actual age and how that intersects with the client's developmental history.

This understanding carries profound implications for therapeutic practice. Therapists must maintain ongoing self-awareness about their own developmental journey and how their changing life circumstances influence the therapeutic dynamic. A therapist who begins their career in their twenties will find that their *transference role* evolves as they age, marry, have children, experience losses, or undergo other life transitions. Each phase of their personal development opens different avenues for client projections while potentially closing others.

The concept extends beyond age to encompass other personal characteristics such as gender, sexual orientation, race, physical appearance, cultural background, and even subtle aspects of personality or communication style. A therapist's visible wedding ring, their manner of dress, their accent, or their office décor all become potential hooks upon which clients hang their unconscious material. The therapeutic relationship thus becomes a complex interplay between the client's internal world and the therapist's actual presence and characteristics.

This perspective challenges therapists to develop what might be called *transference literacy*, the ability to recognize how their own evolving identity contributes to the therapeutic field. Rather than viewing themselves as *blank screens*, therapists are encouraged to understand themselves as active, changing participants whose personal evolution continuously reshapes the therapeutic dynamic. This awareness can enhance their ability to recognize, interpret, and work productively with the transference material that emerges. Therapists need to adopt a nuanced understanding of therapeutic relationships, one that acknowledges the inevitable and valuable ways in which real characteristics of real people, both therapists and clients, create the specific conditions under which unconscious material can emerge, be explored, and potentially be resolved.

The recognition, acknowledgement, and working-through of these elements distinguishes psychoanalytic psychotherapy from other well-intentioned forms of support offered by teachers, aid workers, religious figures, and community leaders. While these helping relationships have value, they lack the specific framework that defines therapeutic practice.

The therapeutic relationship requires the therapist to navigate a delicate balance: maintaining empathic connection with the client through careful listening while preserving sufficient separateness to offer interpretations and suggest new ways of thinking and feeling. This dual position prevents both therapist and client from becoming trapped in the repetitive defensive cycles that originally brought the client to seek help.

Through skilful interpretation and holding by the therapist, both participants can recognize these patterns, *defence mechanisms* that once served a protective function but now constrain the client's capacity for a fuller, more creative existence. The art lies in identifying when these once-necessary defences have become obstacles to growth.

The capacity to recognize the separateness of the other and accept them as they are while simultaneously maintaining a genuine, reciprocal, open, and creative connection embodies what I understand as *ambivalence.* This ambivalence emerges from the coexistence of loving feelings towards the other alongside the acknowledgement and integration of aggressive impulses.

Following Freud, these dual forces, love and aggression, Eros and Thanatos, are conceptualized not as binary opposites locked in eternal conflict but as existing along a dynamic spectrum. Each point on this continuum represents a unique configuration of both elements, reflecting the complex emotional reality of human relationships.

This understanding of ambivalence as an integrated capacity, rather than a pathological state, becomes crucial in therapeutic work, where the ability to hold both loving and aggressive feelings simultaneously allows for authentic engagement without idealization or demonization of the other.

Clearly, when clients first begin therapy they may be far from being at that desired position. Often, it is an aim we strive towards. We may never fully reach it nor stay at that position undisturbed, but we continuously reach out towards such a goal.

We are all born into the care of a primary caregiver, who in the early days and weeks of our lives becomes fully devoted to meeting our essential needs. This profound dedication, which Winnicott termed *primary maternal preoccupation*, represents a crucial psychological state wherein the caregiver's attention becomes almost entirely absorbed by the infant's requirements.

Without this intensive devotion, the infant cannot survive the period of total dependence that characterizes early human development. This phase demands not merely physical care but a quality of attention and responsiveness that enables the infant to begin forming the foundation of psychological security and *epistemic trust* that will inform all subsequent relationships.

Epistemic trust as defined by Peter Fonagy (b. 1952) describes the individual's developmental capacity to trust information communicated by others as accurate, relevant, and personally meaningful. Its roots are in early childhood, based upon a secure attachment and caregiver attunement, which allow for openness to social learning. When epistemic trust is intact, people can learn from each other and adapt flexibly. Stressful life events will lead to epistemic mistrust or hypervigilance, making it difficult to accept help or new knowledge.

Over time, the infant gradually develops capacities that enable movement beyond total dependency. Daniel Stern (1934–2012), in his work *The Interpersonal World of the Infant*, illuminated how infants construct their sense of self through the internalization of sensory, emotional, and cognitive experiences within the relational matrix with their caregivers.

This developmental process unfolds along a dynamic continuum between dependence and autonomy, a fundamental tension that persists throughout the human lifespan. Rather than viewing development as a linear progression from dependence to autonomy, Stern's work reveals how we continuously negotiate our need for connection alongside our drive towards individual identity and agency.

This fundamental dynamic manifests in our capacity for closeness and love alongside our simultaneous need to create a certain distance from the other. In every intimate relationship, whether familial, romantic, friendship, or professional. we experience the coexistence of desires for connection and impulses towards withdrawal or separation.

The experience of aggressive feelings towards those we love represents not a contradiction or pathology but an inherent aspect of *authentic human relationships.* This emotional oscillation constitutes a constant undercurrent in all meaningful connections, reflecting the complex nature of human attachment and the inevitable tensions that arise when individual autonomy meets relational intimacy.

The therapeutic action lies not in eliminating these conflicting impulses but in developing the capacity to recognize, integrate, and consciously navigate them. As we cultivate awareness of this paradoxical holding of love and aggression, we expand our freedom to choose deliberate responses rather than remain captive to unconscious compulsions. This conscious engagement with *ambivalence* transforms potentially destructive patterns into opportunities for deeper understanding and more authentic relationship.

In *a good-enough environment*, one that meets our early needs while establishing appropriate boundaries, we develop into creative, socially engaged individuals capable of forming meaningful relationships while preserving our essential uniqueness. This optimal developmental trajectory allows for the integration of connection and autonomy that characterizes psychological health.

However, when the environment proves inadequate or harmful, emotional development continues along maladaptive pathways. Human development cannot pause or await better conditions; it must proceed regardless of circumstances, adapting to whatever reality presents itself for the sake of the ultimate goal: survival.

The resulting individual and relational maladaptive patterns constitute what we understand as defence mechanisms, i.e. psychological patterns that become essential for both emotional and physical survival, even when causing pain to the individual. These defensive formations represent the mind's ingenious, if sometimes costly, solutions to impossible circumstances.

Even in cases where development appears to have been arrested due to severe trauma, I propose that we are witnessing not stagnation but rather the operation of extraordinarily powerful defensive strategies. These mechanisms aim to safeguard the individual's survival, even when this protection requires encasing the self within what may seem an impenetrable psychological fortress. Such extreme defensive measures, while potentially isolating, represent the mind's determination to preserve the core of the individual against overwhelming threat.

Winnicott's terms of the *true self* and the *false self* conceptualize these areas of the mind as distinct but interconnected. All individuals naturally develop *a false self* structure as a means of protecting their authentic core, the *true self*, from potential harm or overwhelming external demands. In optimal psychological health, these defensive mechanisms remain flexible and adaptive, serving as a protective buffer rather than a rigid barrier. Thus healthy false self allows individuals to navigate social expectations and external pressures while preserving access to their authentic feelings, desires, and creative potential. The key lies in maintaining permeability between these self-states, enabling the person to engage genuinely with the world while safeguarding their essential autonomy and separateness.

When functioning well, this dynamic interplay between true and false self enhances rather than constrains personal freedom, allowing for both social adaptation and authentic self-expression.

Trauma and Loss

Individuals seeking emotional support are burdened with unresolved and uncontained significant losses that have fundamentally shaped their psychological development. These early experiences manifest through various personal and interpersonal *symptoms* that may appear puzzling or self-defeating to outside observers.

These symptoms do not represent moral failings or character defects, as was once commonly believed. Instead, they constitute sophisticated defensive structures that enabled the individual to survive in adverse circumstances where love and aggression remained poorly integrated within their developmental environment. The child internalized these patterns, creating adaptive strategies that while perhaps necessary for survival at the time may now limit their capacity for fulfilling relationships and authentic self-expression.

Understanding symptoms through this lens transforms our therapeutic approach from one of symptom removal to one of recognizing and honouring the individual's creative survival strategies while gently facilitating the development of more flexible and life-enhancing adaptive mechanisms.

When we meet a client in therapy, we experience the entirety of their lived experience, their authentic self interwoven with protective adaptations. The person before us represents a survivor whose psychological defences have enabled them to navigate circumstances that might otherwise have been overwhelming.

Our therapeutic outlook must begin with profound respect for these defensive structures, recognizing their essential role in the client's survival even when they manifest in ways that appear self-defeating or destructive. Each symptom, each seemingly irrational behaviour, each rigid pattern carries within it the wisdom of *adaptation*, however costly that adaptation may have become.

The therapeutic task involves helping clients understand and gradually rework these protective mechanisms that once served as lifelines but now generate the very symptoms that brought them to seek help. This process requires delicate balance: honouring the creative intelligence of their survival strategies while gently facilitating the development of more flexible responses that can serve their current life circumstances. We work not to eliminate defences but to expand the repertoire of adaptive possibilities, allowing for greater freedom, creativity, and authenticity while maintaining the essential protective functions these mechanisms originally served.

Trauma is used nowadays in connection with almost any occurrence that entails fear, pain, and loss. I argue that there has been an inflation in how it is being used and applied to various events. It has taken such a hold in daily language that in a sense we need to extract it from mundane usage and reestablish its significance as a clinical term. I suggest that we need to do that not as a semantic measure but to sharpen our ability to listen to the way it appears in our clients' words and help them regain the sense of *agency* which is lost when trauma really hits the individual.

My main claim is that trauma is primarily *an unconscious event*. I will make the unpopular claim that not every painful or harmful event, nor every loss experienced by an individual as a child or adult, is necessarily traumatic in the sense that trauma is a severe rupture to the mind, causing havoc, sometime irredeemable, to our sense of continuity and agency in the world. We are truly lost in space and time when we are affected by trauma.

We all suffer losses, deprivations, and other instances when we do not get what we want, at best, or are threatened and injured by what we come by, at worst. Such experiences can be very significant, carry many repercussions, and induce pain and a sense of loss but are not necessarily traumatic.

Loss itself can be part of a good-enough developmental process, in which the individual learns to accept and internalize the fact that living in the world does not allow for complete satisfaction and fulfilment of all desires and needs. In this sense, the various losses we experience throughout life help us become mature individuals who can live with reality as it is, not merely as the illusion we wish it were.

However, certain losses occupy a different place in our mind. Losses we were unable to contain or assign subjective emotional, sensory, or cognitive meaning to because they were too overwhelming or occurred at a life stage when we were not yet equipped to deal with them have the potential to become traumatic.

Trauma signifies a profound rupture in the mind, a tearing of the fabric and continuity of human existence. It is an experience that is perhaps impossible to describe in words or any symbolic form because it operates at a preverbal level.

A distressing event that penetrates deep into the primordial layers of development, where language has not yet fully formed, constitutes trauma. Conversely, a painful event or loss that the individual can talk about and describe has a good chance of being integrated into the individual's narrative and not necessarily become traumatic in the sense of that deep emotional rupture.

Of course, the distinction between a traumatic and a non-traumatic event is neither binary nor clear-cut. It is more accurate to think of trauma as existing on a spectrum. Any difficult or painful experience in the present has the potential to become traumatic, even in retrospect, as many survivors of childhood abuse, war veterans, and survivors of the Holocaust can testify. Freud used the term *Nachträglichkeit*, a mode of belated understanding or retroactive attribution of sexual or traumatic meaning to earlier events, to describe this. Chapters Five to Eight provide examples of such instances.

Resilience and the Uncanny

One factor that may render an event traumatic for an individual is their *resilience* prior to the event. Based on the individual's previous experience, if they have been through stressful experience but had a good-enough environment to see them through and support them in real time, the more likely they will be able to cope with difficult events and losses in life without these necessarily penetrating the deepest, most fragile layers of their mind, where they might meet early developmental fissures and become traumatic.

If that resilience is weakened, and the person's defences fail to mitigate the harmful impact of the stressful event, traumatic reverberations may emerge in the unconscious. In this context, it is also significant to consider that the resilience of the individual is sustained by the collective resilience of their community. In societies and communities that are under continuous stress, such as Israel, individuals will find it harder to sustain their personal resilience and are more prone to triggering past traumatic experiences.

It is often argued that Israeli society overall is a society in constant danger of trauma. Having been mostly based on the immigration of Holocaust survivors after World War II, including the Jewish communities from North Africa and other countries who emigrated during the 1950s, having suffered persecution too, it is a society hardened by stress. This does not necessary indicate a greater resilience. As I will discuss in the *two final chapters* of the book, being continuously under existential threat – as Israeli society, Israeli citizens, and Jews around the world have been during so many years – creates collective symptoms ranging from an increased prevalence of PTSD to various forms of reaction formation, often expressed through reactive aggressive behaviours and identification with extreme nationalism.

I believe that one of the factors that can strengthen individual and collective resilience depends on the level of mature ambivalence individuals and communities have towards what they deem dear and what threatens their sense of security. If the individual and the community were to truly acknowledge the complexity of the people and values they hold dear, rather than idealizing or underestimating them and therefore over-reacting to any real or imaginary threat to their existence, their resilience would be higher. They would be better equipped to deal with periods of instability, mild threat, and challenges to the status quo.

An example of such an ambivalence towards an idealized concept can be seen in the reaction to the concept of *home*. This is a central idea in psychoanalysis theories. Winnicott described it best when he referred to *home* as a place where *a facilitating environment* exists, allowing the individual to develop independently and creatively, but also as a place where destructive influences can generate a sense of threat and bring about excessive defensiveness.

Home is also the place that enables the nourishment required for healthy development, but which can also sometimes become a source of toxic nourishment, leading to a pathological internalization of one's self-image and relationships with others, patterns that are then repeated in adult life. Thus, home is indeed our fortress and the place to which we belong, but it can also be the place where we experience our deepest wounds.

The paradoxical role of *home*, as both a place of safety and of potential danger, is captured in Freud's concept of *the uncanny (das Unheimliche)*. Freud used this term to describe the unsettling experience when something deeply familiar also feels strange or threatening. The German word itself reflects this tension: *heimlich* means both homely and hidden, and its opposite, *unheimlich*, reveals what was meant to stay concealed.

Freud explained that in early childhood, *home* is usually experienced as a safe and loving place. Yet moments of conflict with parents can suddenly reveal unexpected sides of them that feel alien or frightening. The secure bond is shaken, and what once felt protective can seem threatening. Melanie Klein described this early stage as *the schizoid-paranoid position*, in which the child splits parents into good and bad figures, unable to see them as whole, complex beings. Only later, in *the depressive position*, does the child begin to accept that love and loss, comfort and frustration, exist together in the same relationship.

This double experience of *home*, both reassuring and unsettling, illustrates the essence of the uncanny. It mirrors the developmental tension between dependence and independence. As children and later adolescents, we gradually move from reliance on parental figures towards separation and autonomy. But this shift is rarely smooth. The familiar bonds of childhood can suddenly feel alien, as our wish for independence brings hostility or estrangement into formerly loving relationships.

In adolescence, this process intensifies with the rediscovery of *sexuality*. Early affectionate bonds with parents, once based on closeness and bodily intimacy, take on new and disturbing meanings under the pressure of puberty. The familiar becomes strange again, and the homely turns uncanny.

If these inner conflicts remain unresolved, the individual may remain split, idealizing the *good* aspects of relationships while rejecting the *bad*. Such unresolved splits make it harder to withstand stress, as crises in life can reactivate old vulnerabilities. For those whose early environment was not *good enough, resilience* is especially fragile, leaving them more exposed to trauma when reality presents challenges.

The Art of Listening to the Traces of Loss

In August 1899, just before publishing his most famous work, *The Interpretation of Dreams*, Freud wrote a letter to Wilhelm Fliess (1858–1928) that captures a profound insight into the nature of human *sexuality*. In it, Freud expressed his growing conviction that everyone is originally bisexual, and that the libido fluctuates between male and female objects depending on life circumstances and inhibitions. He famously wrote that every sexual act is a process involving four individuals.

In the 1899 letter, Freud acknowledges a crucial truth: that every person contains both masculine and feminine elements. This idea reappears in the 1920 edition of the *Three Essays on the Theory of Sexuality*, where he wrote that it is important to regard *bisexuality* as a fundamental fact of human life. In every individual, male or female, the biological disposition probably includes both male and female characteristics.

Understanding human existence as founded upon a natural bisexual structure, one that translates into mental bisexuality, is central to the pluralistic worldview psychoanalysis has gradually embraced. What is often perceived as a binary opposition, male and female, is, from this perspective, better understood as two interwoven aspects of a single whole.

Most individuals ultimately follow one developmental path or the other, leaving behind aspects of the self that do not align with the chosen trajectory. This raises an important question: what happens to the paths not taken? Are they simply abandoned, or do they persist in the unconscious, shaping the mind from beneath awareness?

I suggest that in the human experience, nothing is ever truly lost. What is forgotten, repressed, denied, or even sublimated leaves behind *traces*, residues we can follow through therapeutic work or creative expression. These traces are not limited to sexuality alone. They include all parts of the self that have been left behind, forgotten, or blocked from conscious life.

In this light, the search for such traces becomes another possible answer to the question: *what is it that I do when I do what I do?* In therapy, we strive to recover these lost parts of the self, sometimes reconstructing them anew. By giving voice to these *traces*, by acknowledging, representing, and elaborating them, we allow for richer intrapsychic experience, deeper interpersonal relationships, and more vibrant social engagement.

Thus, the process of therapy can be understood as the search for the *traces* of the parts of us that have been lost, denied, or suppressed, and allowing them creative expression. It is precisely the loss, denial, suppression, and oppression of these parts that underlie much of our psychological pain. Pathological defence mechanisms, distorted patterns of interaction, and limited or harmful modes of self-expression distort those parts. To recover, repair, and rebuild these missing or silenced aspects of the self, we must learn *to listen*, deeply and attentively, to both our clients and ourselves.

I had the great fortune of meeting the Indian psychoanalyst Salman Akhtar (b. 1946) at the 2018 European Federation for Psychoanalytic Psychotherapy (EFPP) conference in Belgrade. There, I was introduced to his remarkable book on the art of listening.

In his book, Akhtar proposes a model of listening structured across four interwoven levels, offering a rich framework for understanding what it truly means to listen in a therapeutic context. He begins by referring to Freud's 1912 paper on therapeutic technique, in which Freud advised analysts to simply listen without worrying about whether the client is consciously hiding something from them. What is truly important, Freud wrote, will be retained through unconscious memory *traces*. This idea mirrors the rule of *free association* on the client's part. Just as the client speaks freely, the therapist listens freely, openly, and without judgement or directive intervention.

In his inspiring study of the therapeutic relationship, Akhtar created a sophisticated account of listening that goes beyond the merely mechanical, revealing instead a nuanced play of human understanding. His four-tiered framework, *objective, subjective, empathic, and intersubjective listening*, constitutes not merely a therapeutic technique, but rather a phenomenological design that allows for a closer approach to what the client says and doesn't say.

Objective Listening emerges as the basic layer, wherein the therapist assumes the role of disciplined observer, maintaining a position of curious neutrality. The therapist assumes an almost forensic position, observing the manifest content of discourse, the client's choice of words and grammatic patterns. This mode demands a kind of bifocal attention: simultaneously engaged yet detached. The therapist becomes an archaeologist of speech, excavating meaning from the deep layers of language; allowing the unconscious text to reveal itself through slips of tongue, peculiar phrasing, and other linguistics expressions that allow glimpses to the underlying layers.

Subjective Listening represents a qualitative shift towards *the hermeneutic*, a movement from observation to interpretation. Here, the therapist's own unconscious becomes a receptive instrument, attuned to the client's unconscious communications. This is listening with what Freud might have called *evenly suspended attention*, yet it transcends mere passivity. The therapist's mind becomes a resonating chamber, vibrating with the client's unconscious expressions. Transference becomes a compass, guiding the therapist towards territories of meaning that resist direct articulation.

Empathic Listening ventures into still more intimate areas, requiring the therapist to contain the client's projective identifications. In this mode, the boundary between self and other becomes permeable without dissolving entirely. The therapist temporarily inhabits the client's inner world, experiencing from within, as it were, their private sense of their emotional reality. This is not mere intellectual understanding, but rather a form of intuitive knowing, a brief excursion into the client's internal landscape where fantasy and reality interweave with equal ontological weight.

Intersubjective Listening represents the most sophisticated, and contentious, form of therapeutic presence, acknowledging that meaning emerges not from either participant alone but from the liminal space between them. The therapeutic dyad becomes a co-creative matrix wherein understanding is perpetually negotiated and renegotiated. Clinical material belongs neither exclusively to client nor therapist but emerges from their mutual enactment, a dialogue of unconscious communications that continuously reshapes both participants. This mode recognizes that interpretation itself is an intersubjective creation arising from the tension between two subjectivities in dynamic exchange.

I find Akhtar's contribution unique and practical in that it articulates a fluid, multidimensional framework that mirrors the complexity of human communication itself. While *objective listening* may serve as the initial structure upon which therapeutic understanding is constructed, the therapist's art is in the capacity to move fluidly between these registers, guided by what Bion called *intuition*, that ineffable capacity to know without knowing how one knows.

This framework acknowledges that *therapeutic listening* is simultaneously archaeological and anticipatory, excavating the past while remaining exquisitely attuned to the emergent present. It is a form of attention that must hold paradox. It must remain engaged yet not too involved, intimate yet with clear ethical boundaries.

Yet Akhtar's model confronts us with an enduring epistemological humility. We must acknowledge that we are ultimately unable to totally understand the singularity of human experience, hard as we try. Each person carries within themselves an inner core, which Christopher Bollas (b. 1943) called *unthought known*, that we must leave unprobed.

Nevertheless, the therapeutic effort persists not in the illusion of complete understanding but in the commitment to ever-more sophisticated forms of recognition. We refine our listening not to achieve perfect comprehension but to honour the complexity of what we cannot fully grasp. In this sense, therapeutic listening becomes an act of epistemic trust.

Listening, then, emerges as both method and ethical principle. It is the basic gesture through which we approach the irreducible otherness of another human being while simultaneously discovering the limits and possibilities of our own capacity for understanding. In Akhtar's hands, listening transcends mere clinical skill to become a form of ethical attention, a way of being present to the world that honours both what can be known and what must remain forever beyond our reach.

This is, indeed, the essence of *what we do when we do what we do*: we listen at the edge of the unknowable, creating spaces where meaning can emerge even as mystery deepens. The art lies not in the elimination of uncertainty but in learning to dwell creatively within it, allowing our refined attention to become a bridge between the solitude of individual experience and the possibility of genuine human contact.

In his sombre yet groundbreaking essay *Beyond the Pleasure Principle* (1920), Freud explored the mind's puzzling tendency to repeat early relational patterns, even when those patterns were traumatic. I would propose that this compulsion to repeat is not solely the result of emotional damage or a pathological loop. It may also express a creative hope: the yearning that this time something different will happen, that the world will respond more adequately to unmet needs.

Through the process of *mourning*, we begin to loosen the grip of the past and create space for new experience. We open ourselves to life's vitality, which Freud called the *life instincts*, and to *sexuality* in its broadest generative sense. While suffering may be inevitable, it need not dominate. *The compulsion to repeat* can become an opening for growth, for healing, for transformation.

This book is dedicated to our shared efforts to repair the wounds borne by individuals and societies around the world. Often, these wounds are inherited, transmitted silently across generations. While we had no voice in how they came to us, we do have the power to respond to them now, with courage and creativity. In choosing to listen, we begin the journey of hope, recovery, and renewal.

Chapter 2

Fiction, Truth, and Authenticity

Navigating the Ethical Borderlands of Therapeutic Writing

While photography and films play important roles in my creative life, writing has been my primary means of expression and remains the medium through which I express what matters most to me.

Since beginning my therapeutic career more than 34 years ago, my writing has increasingly engaged with clinical and theoretical material alongside my ongoing work in prose and poetry. This evolution has led me to wrestle with questions such as: how does my engagement with writing, a formative experience that largely defines my creative identity, influence my work as a therapist and vice versa? When writing fiction and poetry, am I in fact writing about my clinical experience? How can I write about my clinical experience without elaborating it beyond authentic accuracy?

Freud of course was acutely aware of that when he wrote in 1895 that he found it strange that his clinical case studies read like short stories rather than scientific reports. Freud's frustration was with his struggle to establish psychoanalysis as a scientific discipline, a preoccupation which has been haunting the profession ever since. In his first published case studies in 1895, he also confessed to feeling at odds at the mere publication of clinical material as it breached the basic rule of *confidentiality*. He justified doing it nevertheless by the assertion that that was the only way to further his pioneering work. He did it for the sake of scientific progress.

Freud was very good at posing questions that defied clear and permanent answers. Thus, his questions remain valid and still need examining today. The question that relates to the validity of his material as objective scientific data is still debated: was the data he received from dreams, and his clients, scientifically refutable or purely subjective and therefore fictional and not open to scientific probing?

It is only during the last few decades that Freud's claim for the scientific basis of his theories has been given some credence by the likes of the neuropsychoanalyst Mark Solms (b. 1963) and others, who are arguing for instance that Freud's claim regarding the function of dreams as protecting sleep is scientifically sound. The scope of this book does not allow for further exploration of such issues, but one glance at the reading list at the end of the book will provide the avid reader with plenty of material.

DOI: 10.4324/9781003683162-2

The other question is an ethical one and concerns the issue of confidentiality, so pivotal to the therapist–client relationship. The issue of confidentiality draws its roots from medical confidentiality but also from religious models of counselling. Is the therapist permitted under certain circumstances to share what clients tell them in confidence?

In the following pages, I will focus upon the issue of sharing such information through writing. There are of course other forms of possible breaches of that confidence. Sharing information through *supervision* and peer groups is perhaps inevitable, especially during the early stages of one's therapeutic career and during times of clinical uncertainty. Even then, confidentiality must be observed, especially when such sharing with peers is done in professional conventions or other large group settings. The importance of such sharing will be demonstrated in Chapter Four.

The Dangerous Allure of Clinical Material

During my career, I have participated in several thousand therapeutic sessions. After each one, I write notes not merely for legal, ethical, or archival purposes but as an integral part of processing the therapeutic experience itself. This is part of my *reverie* and *working through*. I noticed, particularly with treatments extending beyond a few months, how this writing process deepens my understanding. Week after week, my notes begin forming a narrative. More than once I have thought that what I witness, whether in the client's story, my own thoughts, or the dynamics unfolding between us, could serve as the basis for compelling fiction.

When it comes to sharing with others what clients tell me, beyond areas of supervision as mentioned earlier, I maintain the strictest confidentiality. Any use of therapeutic material outside a professional context constitutes, in my view, a problem concerning the trust clients place in me. Any public use of clinical material, even with direct client involvement and explicit consent, violates a fundamental principle of therapy and might undermine the therapeutic process.

The idea of having to seek consent from the client to do so is already a troubling issue. Due to the inherent imbalance in the power relation in the room, seeking a client's consent is in fact taking advantage of the power relation. The client's ability to give consent to an act which goes beyond their intended goal in coming to therapy is so entwinned in various *transference* issues that exploring them would mean taking the therapy to regions beyond the client's actual needs.

One of the things I always tell my clients at the beginning of the relationship is that they are invited to freely share all their thoughts with me and that they have full confidentiality. Anything short of intention to commit serious crime will remain in the room and not be shared. The clear justification for such a severe rule is that I fear that my ethical integrity and ability to listen will be compromised if I don't adhere to it.

This principle guides my practice absolutely: no client has come to me to have their words shared outside the room. They all seek help because of distress or emotional difficulty, hoping I can help them unravel the complexities they face. Using their words as inspiration for fiction is a problem. As I wrote, the only exception I see as ethically viable and even necessary is during training and at times when the need for peer consultation is clear. When students accept clients for therapy, they are required to share with them that they are in training and therefore are required to be in supervision where they share the details of the therapy. This of course raises another issue when clients express their initial mistrust towards students, fearing that they are getting second rate therapy. In my long career as a supervisor, I have found that in most cases, this initial mistrust, when dealt with openly, dissipates quite quickly, allowing for excellent therapeutic work to take place.

The adherence to the mode of listening I introduced in Chapter One requires that I maintain absolute commitment to confidentiality. Yet, the desire to write creatively and without boundaries remains. Complete denial of that desire also threatens the containment I worked so hard to develop.

Will I become preoccupied with thoughts of the narcissistic sacrifice I am making by giving up my desire to write and publish? There is a real possibility that such thoughts could also impair the quality of my listening just as much as if I were considering my clinical material as fodder for future publication. One could argue that in both cases I would be preoccupied with the fulfilment or denial of my desire, thereby compromising the very quality of listening I strive to maintain.

The solution I propose is not without risks and may not be better than any other solutions, but for me, it offers a reasonable option, particularly when examining the tension between real clinical writing and fictional writing.

In every piece of writing, it is next to impossible to distinguish between subjective and objective elements. For example, an ostensibly objective description of any objective fact which does not own its subjective bias ignores the fact that language is always creative and therefore liable to be a fictional narrative.

I was left with a dilemma. Since writing helps me as a therapist, how do I still engage in writing without betraying the client's trust? I was not prepared to take the path that Freud suggested and use the excuse of scientific need. I had to find a way to allow myself the creative freedom I need to practise my profession while maintaining confidentiality.

As I will demonstrate throughout this book, I have adopted a way of writing about my clinical experience which does not directly involve exposing my clients' stories. This I do by engaging in the theoretical and clinical issues that I am concerned with as well as my own process during my work. What I write about amounts to an elaboration of Freud's *self-analysis*.

Freud was not the first writer to use this confessional method for self-analysis. His objective, though, was unique. His own extensive self-analysis, particularly through *dream analysis* and *free association*, formed the clinical foundation for psychoanalytic theory and laid the framework for the actual practice of psychotherapy as a method to help people with stress, and not just as philosophical confessional investigation.

The practice of self-analysis requires approaching unconscious material that, by definition, resists conscious awareness. Freud recognized this paradox: how can one analyse what remains hidden from oneself? His solution involved paying attention to slips of tongue, dreams, and seemingly irrational thoughts as windows into unconscious processes. Through disciplined attention to these phenomena, he mapped his own emotional landscape, identifying childhood memories, repressed desires, and defensive patterns.

Self-analysis has its limitations. While it remains crucial for self-awareness, the risk of self-deception, bias, and circular reasoning make purely solitary analysis problematic. That is why I am not advocating it as a substitute for therapy or supervision, but rather as the platform for a possible solution to the dilemma I presented earlier. It is a solution to the problem of continuing writing and even publishing insights from clinical work without breaching confidentiality.

Psychoanalysis and Literature: Fiction and Reality

As well as self-analysis, Freud used numerous literary examples to illustrate the clinical theories he developed, thereby recognizing literature as a source of inspiration for those theories. He used an ostensibly objective analysis of literary subjects to demonstrate his clinical discoveries. Writing about his experience and literature served him as a platform through which he explored and developed the psychoanalytic field.

The relationship between writing and psychoanalysis is not as an *objective* investigation of a *subject*, but rather of two equal *subjects* engaging in a study of existential issues, siblings. As Shoshana Felman (b. 1942) wrote, both disciplines conduct this exploration through language, both written and spoken. Such a view of the two disciplines rests on the assumption that the relationship between *objective data* and *subjective fiction* is not so clear. In his review of literary works and their authors' biographies, the Israeli philosopher Avi Sagi (b. 1953) suggests that the biographical story seems to refer to the facts of the writer's life, whereas the fictional story refers to the written expressions of their consciousness. But this contradiction loses its validity when we consider that even an autobiographical story is a fictional story by virtue of being a story that uses language to represent memory. Every choice to include one story or another in an autobiography involves an act of creating fiction and forming narratives that were not necessarily present in the reality of the story as it occurred. The moment we recount something about the past, our consciousness forms a narrative, and thus a fictional element is introduced.

The clinical reality we describe is intersubjective and crucially dependent on our consciousness as therapists when we write about it. Remembering is not a mechanical process of copying the client's words and the therapeutic process into empty cognitive containers. Every act of remembering is a creative act of the person remembering it. Therefore, even writing what is ostensibly factual about therapy is fictional because it stems from the therapist's consciousness. The question of its veracity cannot be determined by external criteria but should be judged by its internal consistency and faithfulness to the principles it is based on. I therefore propose that the *authenticity* of my case studies can be assessed only by the consistency of the subjective data it reveals, not by external scientific-objective standards.

Authenticity is therefore the concept through which we can critically assess how clinical writers describe their therapeutic experiences. Writing fictional but authentic case studies, as I propose to share throughout this book, is an act of interpretation. Since my memory already contains thousands of therapeutic hours, my writing is saturated with them. The process of fictional clinical writing is a reconstruction of *traces* that I assemble from my consciousness, but I also recognize that a lot of content seeps in from my unconsciousness. It is perhaps more revealing of my own process than the processes of my clients.

The details in any clinical account can be viewed as representing an authentic version of what takes place in therapy. When a clinical case study is written based on the details of the case, it is written based on the therapist's memory and thus is an expression of the therapist's consciousness, rather than a one-to-one transcription. It is of course real but represents just a version of the truth. Since it is impossible to reproduce what had taken place in the session, each account of the session would be as fictional and creative as another account, different as it may be.

We cannot be scientific and objective in the accounts of our work, given that the basis of science is the ability to place our assumptions to scientific scrutiny, like repeating the experiment (session) under the same conditions. If the data (session) cannot be repeated (tested) again, it cannot be subjected to scientific scrutiny. The question as to whether science itself is an objective method of inquiry is of course an open one but far beyond the scope of this book.

Authenticity, Play, and Truth

Winnicott's idea of *play* is a crucial element to understanding the elusive nature of what goes on in therapy. Play is an innate human capacity and not, as Freud seems to have suggested, *a sublimation* of aggression. The capacity *to play* emerges as a natural consequence of a *good-enough environment* which allows the child's creativity to flourish within clear boundaries. Winnicott suggested that it develops as a *transitional phenomenon* whereby the child is still undetermined as to the clear distinction between fantasy and reality, between what is theirs and what isn't, between what is coming from within and what is external to his being.

Being able to be in such a fluid imaginative state of mind allows the child's creativity to flourish. It is this creativity that forms the basis for the individual sense of autonomy and freedom. Being in that paradoxical state of mind where one's imagination is allowed to roam allows one to be creative. It is within such a playful state of mind that I propose to read the fictional case studies I shall present.

It does not describe a single client nor a cluster of clients. It is composed of a rich *synchronic* tapestry of clinical details, autobiographical associations, and cultural references woven into my memory over the years. Its writing process is like that of any fictional story. Perhaps it is impossible to decide what is real in it, and what is fictional, except to say that it is entirely real in that it expresses my consciousness, and entirely fictional in that I created it in writing. It represents the therapeutic space in which I work, and at the same time also represents the inner space in which I imagine, as I will demonstrate in the following clinical study of Menachem.

During one of our weekly sessions, Menachem, a 62-year-old man, posed a question that seemed to emerge from the depths of decades-old pain: *"how can I go back to the home I left?"*

After a deliberate pause, he continued:

> *I want to return to the home I abandoned when I was 23. I ran away from my past, from my father, from Israel itself, after the first Lebanon War in 1982. I thought I was escaping him, but now I understand I was running from myself. Is return even possible? My father is dead. How do I go back now? How do I return to say I'm sorry, to tell myself that only now I realize I wasn't fleeing him but from the parts of myself I couldn't face?*

Menachem had entered therapy after months of persistent panic attacks that began following a visit to Israel in 2010. He had spent almost two decades in Amsterdam, building a family and a successful business career. On the surface, he had created a stable life far from the homeland he had fled as a young man. His decision to return was precipitated by a family crisis: his wife's extramarital relationship with another woman had shattered the foundation of his carefully constructed world.

Yet his homecoming only deepened existing fractures. His three daughters, born and raised in Holland, remained there, though they maintained close contact to Israel through frequent visits. Menachem found himself caught between worlds: neither fully Dutch nor fully Israeli, neither the young man who had fled nor the older man who had returned. He carried the weight of unresolved grief for a father he could no longer reach.

At our first session, I met a man who seemed older than his years. His hair was grey, his body lean and stringy. What struck me most was his gaze: direct, penetrating, unwavering. Very typically Israeli. He shook my hand with force, holding that intense eye contact. The gesture lingered in my awareness.

I noticed something unexpected stirring within me, mild hostility in response to what should have been a simple, friendly greeting. The handshake felt less like a greeting and more like a gauntlet thrown down: firm, unrelenting, almost aggressive. And yet, beneath the challenge, I sensed desperation, like the grasp of a drowning man. The thought unsettled me. I knew that reaching someone drowning carries double danger: you may fail to save them, and you may be pulled under yourself.

The session took on the quality of a challenge from the very start, like two roosters testing dominance. I was nearly 20 years younger, yet felt an immediate, primitive urge to assert control in the therapeutic space meant to be mine to hold. Beneath that instinct, though, lay something more familiar: the mix of authority and vulnerability older male figures often evoked in me. I noted this internal shift with both recognition and dread, aware that my own history was already contributing to the encounter. Still, the work had to begin.

In the early sessions, Menachem laid out the complexity of his life. He carried deep anger towards his wife for her betrayal. Though their relationship had known ups and downs, he was shocked to discover her infidelity. He thought that despite difficulties she still saw him as her partner. He was proud of their shared role as parents to three talented, creative daughters. Blaming himself for not seeing the betrayal, he experienced it as a devastating blow to his self-esteem. His wound was so deep that he refused to speak with her about anything beyond parenting. He wanted a divorce quickly and was furious that she resisted, insisting on repairing the relationship. For him, trust was broken beyond repair. Returning to Israel felt like the only way to protect himself; living near her was unbearable. The pain triggered panic attacks, for which he began medication.

Once I acknowledged my own transference, I could listen more freely. All I had to do was witness Menachem's story and occasionally offer questions to shape its frame. I felt like a spectator at a play written by a gifted playwright. It was difficult not to admire his storytelling. Menachem noticed my attention and used it. The handshake that had first felt like a cry for help now seemed like an invitation to bear witness to a heroic figure recounting his fall from grace.

My presence as a witness became a supporting role in his effort to restore that heroic image. I even felt proud that such a strong, paternal figure had chosen to lean on me. I didn't yet understand how, but I suspected these dynamics would eventually echo his relationship with his father.

The Hero with a Thousand Faces

After that session, I found myself drawn to Campbell's *The Hero with a Thousand Faces.* Joseph Campbell (1904–1987) explores ancient myths centred on the hero figure, one who embarks on literal and emotional journeys to confront the depths of his mind, overcome profound challenges, and emerge transformed. Campbell draws from mythical figures like *Prometheus* stealing fire from the gods, *Jason* escaping the dragon that guards the golden fleece, and *Aeneas* descending into the underworld to commune with his father's spirit.

I was also reminded of the *rite of passage* that the anthropologist Victor Turner (1920–1983) describes: *separation, initiation*, and *return*. He described *liminal stages* as the middle phase in rites of passage, where people leave one state of life but have not yet entered the next. In this in-between time, old roles are gone, but new roles are not yet fixed. Turner called it a space of uncertainty, ambiguity, and transformation. People may feel lost but also free from normal rules. He argued that this stage allows for creativity and renewal, since social structures loosen. Once the ritual ends, participants re-enter society with new roles, identities, or status, shaped by what they experienced in liminality.

As I reflected on these myths and their interpretations, I recognized a pattern. These existential journeys represent critical stages in the process of separating from the primal experience of *home* as part of the journey to establish an autonomous identity. A recurring feature in many myths is a man engaging with *the feminine*: sometimes she appears as the desired object the hero must win, other times as an obstacle to overcome.

Menachem's story began to feel like a rite of passage: his departure from Israel, forming a new life in Europe, the devastating betrayal, and his painful return. I saw him as a hero struggling with strange, ambiguous events in his descent into the underworld of betrayal.

His powerful handshake from our first session suddenly aligned with this emerging narrative now appeared to be an initial confrontation. It was overcharged with masculine intensity, and perhaps was an expression of Menachem's internal struggle with his father? I recalled Freud's definition of the hero as someone who has dared to rebel against his father and ultimately defeated him.

I arrived at our next session preoccupied, and perhaps burdened, with these literary parallels, carrying an uncomfortable guilt that I might be more absorbed in the literary aspects of the case than in Menachem himself. Was my fascination with potentially writing about this case distracting me from truly listening? I questioned my therapeutic capacity, wondering how helpful I could be while caught in these theoretical webs.

As therapy progressed, Menachem reclaimed a measure of agency. He realized he could no longer ignore his wife's persistent attempts at reconciliation.

She was planning to fly to Israel. After weeks of refusing contact, he confronted an uncomfortable uncertainty: did she want to reconcile because her affair had ended, or did she really want to heal their marriage because she realized her mistake?

The first possibility stirred anger; the second triggered hope. What tormented him most wasn't betrayal itself but its nature. The fact that his wife had chosen a woman as her lover pierced deeper than infidelity. It felt like an assault on his identity as a man.

"If it had been some young, attractive guy, I could understand that", he said with bewildered pain. *"I've thought about that myself, about younger women at work, at events. But a woman? Why a woman?"*

Together we explored this. A younger male rival would have triggered familiar insecurities: jealousy over aging, questions of diminishing appeal, the predictable wounds of middle-aged masculinity. But his wife's choice of a woman shattered that framework. It wasn't about his insufficiency; it implied irrelevance. Her turn towards a woman felt like a rule change that invalidated not just their marriage but his very assumptions about desire, attraction, and his place in the world.

Soon after, Menachem arrived for a session with his familiar intensity. His wife had come to Israel, and they had met. The meeting was painful but transformative. She appeared warm and loving. Though she admitted that traces of her feelings for the other woman remained, she believed they would not endure. She wanted to try again.

For the first time in weeks, Menachem felt he was on a new path. His panic attacks soon receded, likely also due to the medication he had begun before starting therapy. He still felt angry and hurt, but he admitted he remained deeply attached to his wife and wanted to heal together.

Reflecting, he recognized how betrayal had forced him into exile, not by choice but necessity. He could not stay in their European home with wounds so fresh. Yet paradoxically, his return to Israel, his homeland, felt like exile too, awakening estrangement. Now, with reconciliation in sight, he sensed he had emerged from a dark underworld, aided by her forgiving and remorseful presence.

Searching for One's Own Idiom

I couldn't help wondering if my literary reading of Menachem's journey, his descent into an underworld to confront a feminine figure whose betrayal ultimately brings revelation, was entirely coincidental. What was my role in this heroic narrative?

Menachem's descriptions of returning to Israel fascinated me. He recounted how everything felt for him uncanny, simultaneously familiar and alien. He reconnected with family and friends, revisited landscapes from his past, and experienced emotional flashbacks, yet the strange-familiar sensation persisted.

In trying to understand my therapeutic role, I found myself thinking of Freud's concept of *the uncanny*, which I already referred to as a key concept in Chapter One, and which will recur throughout this book.

I sensed that Menachem's complex feelings pointed towards unresolved conflicts we hadn't yet explored in therapy. Should my role be to confront these depths, to stir up old ghosts, or should I be content with our current success, the alleviation in his anxiety symptoms, and his renewed willingness to engage with his wife?

In the following sessions, Menachem continued sharing positive developments in their renewed intimacy. They had decided to visit Israel more often and had even contemplated a return once their daughters complete their studies in Holland. He could manage his business remotely and welcomed the possibility. He informed me we had only a few sessions remaining before concluding therapy as they were returning to Holland. This was well before COVID-19 and the emergence of Zoom meetings.

On the surface, I had reason for satisfaction. Yet I carried an uneasy feeling, as if our work had addressed primarily the surface level and addressed a *screen memory* rather than the unconscious content beneath it. I noticed my thoughts repeatedly turning to Freudian theory. While this wasn't unusual for me, there was something more urgent, more intimate about how these concepts now presented themselves. I wondered if I was turning to Freud as a father figure to help me navigate this critical therapeutic juncture.

I came to sense that a unique language had developed between Menachem and me. This led me to Bollas's *idiom*, an idea I will use extensively throughout this book. Christopher Bollas suggests in the opening page of *Forces of Destiny* that every individual and relationship develop their own distinctive language, essential for sharing unconscious, *unthought known* experiences. He traces this level of language to the primal communication patterns between mother and infant that form basic templates that seek expression in later relationships. This idiom, he proposes, creates the intimacy necessary for authentic communication. The idiom is the articulation of the essence of the individual which is allowed to be expressed given the good-enough parenting environment. In some ways, it is a variation on the *true self* term that Winnicott used. But it differs from it in at least one significant sense. The moralizing true/false dichotomy is absent. Instead, the concept of language is portrayed as a crucial platform through which human articulation is performed. Bollas' idiom is a quality, potential, or aspect of the individual that is hidden within him as a secret script waiting to be discovered.

The question remained: had Menachem and I developed our idiom sufficiently to address what lay beneath the surface of his heroic return, or would we conclude with the restoration achieved, leaving deeper mysteries unexplored?

When Therapist and Client Share a Similar Wound

Menachem had told me about his relationship with his father, who had died a decade earlier. His father was a Holocaust survivor who had escaped the concentration camps by wandering through European forests and joining partisan groups. He arrived in Israel aged 19 and soon after joined the Israeli Defence Forces (IDF) during the War of Independence in 1948, participating in every major conflict since, through to the Yom Kippur War in 1973. Despite experiencing numerous combative events, he seemingly remained unaffected by them outwardly.

Menachem described his father as tough in business and social interactions but gentle with him, though always carrying demanding expectations for achievement. Over the years, they only had a few conversations which went beyond daily necessities. Menachem's attempts to learn about his father's past were usually dismissed. What he knew filtered through his mother's stories.

Reflecting on these fragments Menachem had shared, I began to wonder if his connection with his father was the unconscious content I sensed hovering beneath the surface, masked by the explicit narrative about his wife's betrayal. Initially, I couldn't detect a clear connection, but I suspected that if there was truth to this intuition, it would eventually emerge.

While recounting a conversation about her infidelity, Menachem suddenly burst out: *"It's all because of this damn country. You invest so much in it, and what do you get in return? Nothing! Just more and more demands. Believe me, I won't stay here one more unnecessary moment"*.

The words startled me. They didn't match his usual attitude towards Israel or our present context. My expression must have betrayed my surprise because he laughed: *"Surprised you, didn't I? It surprised me too. But it's something my father used to say"*.

Later in the session, he mentioned that he had planned to visit his father's grave two days earlier but hadn't managed it. That night, he had a terrifying dream about climbing a high cliff, clinging to crumbling rock, and being in mortal danger of falling. He woke as he felt himself slip, plunging into the abyss.

A heavy silence followed. His face was more tormented than I had ever seen it. *"Do you think it's related to my father?"* he asked.

Anything I might say felt banal. I simply acknowledged his feelings. The dream seemed to express what the cemetery visit had stirred. When I asked him to reflect further, he claimed at first he had nothing to say. After silence, he told me again, this time with unusual tenderness, that he had never truly said goodbye to his father.

His father had died suddenly of cardiac arrest in his sleep. Living abroad, Menachem flew in only for the funeral. He carried regret and grief for months, guilty for living so far and for such infrequent contact. That guilt was mixed with anger at his father, whom he blamed for his exile.

"All those years he told us Israel was a damned country, a land that devours its inhabitants. 'I came here because the Nazis murdered my family. But you, stay in Europe. It's better there.'"

He recalled how, during the mourning process over his father, he had struggled to function within his family. His daughters were still young, leaving the burden to his wife. He woke up screaming from nightmares that disturbed her sleep. After a year without improvement, he moved into his study, sleeping there for months. Only later, he realized, did the distance between him and his wife begin. The session ended early; he wanted to speak with her about this.

Two weeks later, Menachem and his wife returned abroad, and therapy ended. Our last two sessions felt strangely anticlimactic. He told me his wife confirmed his insight: his withdrawal after his father's death had widened the distance between them. But Menachem himself seemed already elsewhere. Therapy no longer felt relevant; he felt better and hopeful about renewal.

He thanked me warmly and promised to contact me during future visits to Israel. His gratitude was sincere, yet I was left with lingering doubt. Had we reached true transformation, or had Menachem regained just enough stability to carry on? The question remains unresolved, like the unfinished goodbye to his father.

Epilogue

I felt somewhat inadequate as a psychoanalytic psychotherapist. Though I should have felt pleased with the positive changes in my client's life, I felt those changes had little to do with what I believed was supposed to be happening in therapy. I felt like a CBT therapist.

I know that planned endings, especially good endings, often only occur in films, especially ones made in Hollywood. Life is far more complex, abrupt, and unpredictable. Often, meaning and significance must be dressed upon what actually happens. Shrugging one's shoulders seems the most common and adequate response to questions like I was asking myself regarding how this client was helped by me.

Gaining satisfaction from one's work as a therapist is really nothing like a carpenter's work, as an example. We remain with no concrete bench, table, or sculpture we can appreciate after our work is done. We are left with memories and questions, at best.

Writing therapeutic tales, such as this one, is one way of leaving something concrete to ponder and consider after the client has left. Months later, as I reflected on my own search for paternal guidance in navigating the therapeutic relationship with Menachem, I recognized something which showed me some of the creative aspect of my therapeutic work: my search mirrored his own process and expressed a version of a struggle with a paternal figure that I had sensed from our very first handshake.

At the time, I was deeply engaged in writing my Ph.D. about Lawrence Durrell, the exiled British author whose search for homeland resonated with questions I was exploring in my own life. Durrell's story fascinated me. He was born in India to Anglo-Indian parents but sent at age 12 to boarding school in distant England so he could acquire the formal education necessary to become *the real Brit* his father envisioned. Durrell wrote extensively about this defining experience, both overtly and in veiled references, describing it as the *secret wound* of his life. Throughout his subsequent wanderings, he found himself drawn to paternal figures from whom he hoped to gain direction, inspiration, and recognition. I will return to my work on his novels and the inspiration he gave me in Chapter Nine.

In some ways, my work with Menachem helped me along my own journey as an individual seeking to trace the footpaths of a hero, or rather a protagonist, I have adopted, Lawrence Durrell, in my own descent into the underworld, and back. Menachem of course will never know this, but I thank him silently from time to time.

The fictional tale of Menachem is not just a case illustration but a testament to the profound ethical labyrinth that every therapist must navigate. His story, or rather the story I have constructed from the subjective layers of countless therapeutic sessions, illuminates the fundamental tension between the therapist's duty to maintain confidentiality and exclusivity and the human need to transform experience into meaning through narrative.

In crafting this fictional composite, I hope I showed that the boundary between authenticity and fabrication dissolves into something more nuanced: a creative loyalty to emotional truth that goes beyond quasi-scientific accuracy. Menachem's heroic descent into the underworld of betrayal, his confrontation with paternal ghosts, and his emergence into renewed possibilities address universal patterns of human behaviour as signposts on the road to recovery.

Menachem's quest for reconciliation with his father's legacy and my own scholarly pursuit of Lawrence Durrell's exiled wanderings reveal how therapeutic sessions become mutual creations of meaning. The therapist, in bearing witness to the client's narrative, inevitably discovers reflections of their own unresolved themes, discovering a shared language born from the interplay of two humans seeking understanding.

Ethical clinical writing maintains the therapist's subjectivity and allows its conscious integration. Through fictional reconstruction, it is possible to honour the client's trust and the creative drive without violating the confidentiality.

Chapter 3

Threshold Encounters

The Paradox of Beginnings in Psychoanalytic Psychotherapy

Sue, a 31-year-old Philippian woman working as a carer for a disabled elderly woman in Israel, recently experienced a miscarriage. She has been in Israel for only two months and speaks little Hebrew. She arrives at a special unit of the local welfare services in Jerusalem dedicated to supporting migration workers, accompanied by her brother, who is also a migrant worker. Both are working legally in Israel, so they have access to medical and welfare services.

When does therapy begin? Is it when the client enters the room? Is it when the client begins to speak? Is it when they are referred or arrive to the first meeting? Or is the beginning in the therapist's mind, when they first start thinking about the client, the moment of conception?

This chapter will explore in some depth the first session of psychotherapy. I place particular significance on the first session not out of determinism but rather as I believe that striving to understand how things begin helps in the task I have established in Chapter One of *listening to the traces* of the parts that have been repressed, denied, or forgotten. This search continues throughout the course of therapy and even if an analysis of the first session does not yield significant traces, we should not assume that the therapy has gone off course. In that sense, each beginning of each future session is a repetition of that very first session, and we are given the chance, due to *repetition compulsion*, to begin anew. True to what I have established in Chapter Two, I shall use fictional clinical material to illustrate my arguments.

As transpired later, Sue was two months pregnant when she arrived in Israel but was not aware of it. She only discovered her pregnancy when she was rushed to hospital, having fainted during work, and there she discovered she was undergoing a miscarriage. After being discharged from the hospital, she had felt depressed, lacked appetite and motivation, and had trouble sleeping. She hadn't disclosed to anyone the circumstances in which she conceived and was reluctant to discuss the matter with anyone. Her brother too was reticent about it even though their friends suspected he knew more than he divulged.

DOI: 10.4324/9781003683162-3

Though they were satisfied with her work, the people she worked with had agreed to continue employing her only if she sought help from the welfare services, as they feared for her health.

After filling in some online forms, Sue was referred to a social worker named Shelly.

> *At the local welfare services, Sue finds Shelly's door closed and gently knocks. A voice calls from inside the room:*
>
> *"I will come to you shortly. Wait outside".*
>
> *Sue does not understand the meaning and opens the door. Shelly looks up and says sharply,*
>
> *"I told you to wait outside!"*
>
> *Sue retreats to the waiting room. She may not have understood the words properly, but the tone of voice was clear.*
>
> *A few minutes later, Shelly calls out from the room and invites Sue in. Sue had felt intimidated by Shelly's tone and hesitates. Seeing that, Shelly smiles at her and makes a welcoming gesture. Sue gets up and walks slowly into the open room, glancing back at her brother in the waiting room.*

Starting off on the Wrong Foot

Even without going into a deeper analysis of these details, it is safe to say that such a beginning does not clearly indicate to the anxious client that they are welcome. It does not create the necessary initial atmosphere where *epistemic trust* might begin to evolve. It is a failure in containment, though a minor one, and the informed psychoanalytic psychotherapist will need to pause to understand its unconscious origins and glean ways of responding in order to repair the situation so that the course of therapy does not go astray.

It is, in some ways, like giving birth to a child with special needs. The parents need to adjust themselves quickly, deal with their sense of *mourning*, and find ways to respond to the newborn's needs. The baby that has arrived may not be the baby they have wished for and imagined, but it is the baby that they need to take care of. Without trying to sound too dramatic or harsh, one could say that to be able to take care of the baby the parents need to be able *to mourn* the baby that they will not have.

Such a beginning is akin to meeting the experience of *death* early on, well before one is ready to do so. Something begins and its fragility reminds us that it might end as quickly as it began. In this sense, a beginning is *the beginning of the end*. The informed therapist holds that thought in their mind as they enter a new therapeutic situation.

The end of therapy, like the end of life, is always a surprise, an event that we may prepare ourselves for but will always catch us off guard. One's ability to hold that thought in mind helps, I believe, to start off the therapy journey on safer grounds. One needs to begin therapy with the inevitability of its end always in mind. Therefore, every moment counts. I believe that the attitude the therapist needs to strive towards is that of *evenly suspended attention* as Freud termed it or *unconditional acceptance*, as Carl Rogers (1902–1987) phrased it. Such an attitude is often mistaken for neutrality or distance, but it is not that. It is the ability to acknowledge whatever happens without trying to judge it, re-direct it, or deny its existence, even when unpleasant. In other words, to be able to accept life in its fullness, the therapist also needs to acknowledge death and its vicissitudes, including the kind of *empathic failures* as displayed by Shelly.

The beginning of the therapeutic process is one of the crucial moments in psychoanalytic therapy. It is like the birth of the therapeutic process. The location of such a meeting can be the municipal social welfare office, a corridor in a hospital, a room in a mental health clinic or at probation services, or the social worker's room in residential institutions.

In all cases, the first session between therapist and client is the foundation of the therapeutic relationship and often serves as a microcosm of the entire process. The informed therapist needs to plan and prepare for this meeting.

The first session is never just an assessment interview or a getting-to-know-you meeting. It is always conducted under a certain tension stemming from the client's anxiety about stepping into the unknown and, to some extent, the therapist's anxiety. The therapist's capacity to contain this tension will determine the client's ability to open up and bring forth whatever brought them to the meeting.

The client's anxiety may seem more understandable, as they are the one seeking help. However, the therapist's anxiety also plays a significant role, as they are now placed in a position where they must address both conscious and unconscious wishes for help. These wishes place pressure on the therapist, who naturally wants to respond professionally and humanely. The therapist's intention is to help, but to do so effectively they must adhere to certain *professional boundaries.* This might create tension between the *formal aspects* of the meeting such as– time management, privacy, and the level of concrete help offered, and the *informal aspects* such as unconditional acceptance and empathy.

Every first meeting between a therapist and a client is between two people who until that moment were total strangers. Therefore, it's difficult to expect an open conversation in which at least one of them shares their emotional difficulties straight away. However, that is exactly what begins to happen as the session unfolds. This initially awkward beginning slowly evolves into an intimate meeting. Without this transformation, which does not make void the formal elements such as time management, a therapeutic process cannot truly occur. If this transformation fails, therapy may not proceed, and sessions may end prematurely.

Intimacy is a word mostly used in other contexts such as friendships, amongst family members, and in romantic situations. The therapy dyad does share characteristics with all these social contexts, but it is the crucial *formal aspect* of the relationship which differentiates it as a therapeutic relationship rather than a social one. Perhaps the special therapeutic intimacy is better understood if it is seen within the *epistemic trust* that needs to be established. As will be expanded upon in Chapter Six, epistemic trust is the individual's ability to trust the information communicated by others as accurate, relevant, and personally meaningful.

Even when such trust and intimacy are attained, the therapeutic relationship will always retain its awkwardness, beyond the natural *ambivalence* discussed in Chapter One, because of its formal aspects. Those formal aspects also guard it from turning into something it was not meant to be. The therapist and client will never become friends, for instance, though they might of course feel very affectionate towards one another and may know one another better than anyone else.

Even when sufficient intimacy and trust are achieved to enable therapy, the therapeutic relationship remains, at its core, a formal relationship: the therapist provides a service, and the client seeks help. The paradox does not disappear; it continues to exist. Trying to dissipate the paradox by breaking the rules constitutes an ethical problem. As I will expand upon in Chapters Four and Five, maintaining those ethical boundaries is crucial.

I think of the beginning of therapy through a developmental model, analogous to the beginning of life. The initial formation of the therapeutic bond lays the groundwork for the entire relationship. Just as we think of the first years of life as shaping the most significant patterns of one's personal and social functioning, so too do the first therapeutic experiences form the foundation for the unfolding process.

As already mentioned, this might give the impression that everything is predetermined, as people often think about psychoanalytic psychotherapy. If therapy begins poorly, as Sue's situation might suggest, it may seem doomed to fail. But that is not necessarily the case.

I will describe in some detail the many processes that I think are at play here. I might be accused of looking too closely, but my experience over the years has taught me that you can never look too closely at the beginning. What seems to be a faulty beginning often turns out to contain valuable information that should not be ignored, for the sake of doing it right. It just requires patience and the willingness to look over the details time and time again.

Every beginning is accompanied by a certain level of anxiety. This anxiety is not necessarily resistance to therapy but rather a natural response to the unknown. Whatever the nature of the client's issues is, their anxieties will be experienced as a threat once entering the therapeutic setting.

Even if the beginning seems full of difficulties, recognizing that they mainly stem from mutual anxiety allows us to manage that anxiety and use it as motivation for the process. The difficulty at the outset is an expression of the client's distress. A therapist who recognizes and contains this difficulty has already taken a significant step towards creating a meaningful connection. The very ability to be open to the client's anxiety and feel its emotional intensity is a sign that the therapist is creating internal space for the client, a space where the anxiety can be transformed.

If this anxiety is understood as fear of getting in touch with painful emotional content, we can work with it rather than denying or suppress it. However, passively accepting this anxiety is not enough. To transform it into a therapeutic engine, the therapist must make conscious efforts to understand what is happening.

As we compare the beginning of therapy to the beginning of life, we can view the client's anxiety as akin to that of a newborn entering the world and expecting a parental figure will be there to receive them. Partial absence of such a figure, or if that figure is emotionally unavailable, will exert overwhelming sensory pressure on the baby. Similarly, without a containing therapeutic presence at the beginning, the client may feel intense emotional pressure, potentially harming their ability to engage with the external world and retreating into themselves as a protective measure.

This initial anxiety is inevitable and signals the possibility of a meaningful experience. This primary anxiety will never disappear completely, and its ongoing presence serves as a reminder of the paradox: therapy is both a formal and intimate process. Acknowledging the existence and legitimacy of this anxiety allows us to engage with it directly, without disguising or denying it.

Hanging On

One of the components that can help the therapist handle and understand the emotional pressure generated by the initial anxiety of therapy is by holding on to the core belief of *hope*.

Hope is not the same as the illusion that the therapist will definitely be able to help the client resolve their issues. Such promises cannot be made, explicitly or implicitly. For the core value of hope to be genuine and not such an illusion of omnipotence, it needs to stem from the therapist's life experience and reliance on their professional experience. The therapist needs to know what they are doing, not in the sense of total control but rather from the creative position of having answers to the question, *what is it that I do when I do what I do.*

The therapist can offer the experience of *hope* to the client only if they are hopeful in their own capacities as therapists, despite the fact they cannot be certain that the outcome will be as desired. They must be hopeful in the sense that they know what they are doing. And when they do not know what they are doing, as I demonstrate in the various case studies in this book, they have a theoretical and experiential foundation from which they derive inspiration. Their constant and creative engagement with the professional core principles that inform their work will give rise to their sense of hope in being good-enough therapists.

Hope is rooted in the therapist's capacity to create *a facilitating space* where the client can feel safe enough to trust the therapist with their pain. By hanging on to hope, the therapist signals to the client that their willingness to listen is based on a readiness to embark on an intersubjective journey that may lead to positive change in the client's life circumstances.

Even in cases where the beginning of therapy is not experienced as positive, and more despair is experienced than hope, we need still to work out what went on, what was being repeated, so we can address it. Hope is not about seeking miracles but rather the opposite. We must remember that we are not trying to reach the ultimate truth but rather to discover *authenticity*.

Feeling hopeful is a strategy that paradoxically connects us to reality, since it shows the gap between wishes and what reality can provide and suggests that we need to maintain our position as listeners without getting overly engaged. Maintaining the paradoxical hopeful and non-engaged position was referred to by Freud as *evenly suspended attention*.

This position has often been misinterpreted and ridiculed as neutrality and detachment, but it is anything but that. The ability to remain in such a position is the most receptive, accepting, and confirming position one can hold to allow someone else to explore the depths of their mind.

The question of whether the ability to offer *hope* is fundamentally grounded in an experience of *love* is an inevitable one. Is it true to say that without love for the client therapy is not possible?

To answer this, we would of course need to fully define what *love* is, a task beyond the scope of this book. I have come to regard the common use of the word *love* as vacuous, requiring much elaboration in order to clarify its ontological significance rather than an empty, demonstrative verb, often concealing repressed and denied emotions. I find it far more practical to think that what we mean by *love* is the innate but also acquired human capacity to *care* for another human being as much and at times more than ourselves. I am inspired in this by the Old Testament phrase *Love your neighbour as yourself* from Leviticus 19:18.

This can be read as an ethic of *empathy*: imagining oneself in the position of another. Love is not simply avoiding harm but actively willing good for others at the same level as for oneself. It can also inspire social justice movements, interfaith dialogue, and humanitarian ethics, as I will discuss in Chapters Ten and Eleven. It functions as a variant of the Golden Rule, appearing in many cultures in similar form. Finally, it establishes that one cannot love another without healthy self-regard.

I propose that the experience of love, essential to hope, is indeed necessary at the beginning of therapy, akin to the good-enough mother's love for her newborn. A good-enough mother is one who can give herself fully to enable the infant's survival and development. I believe that that was what Winnicott meant by *primary maternal preoccupation*.

A measure of *love* is therefore a given that we must assume existed at the start of every person's life. Any person who has survived the first days of life, days marked by complete dependence on the unconditional care of a parental figure, has experienced good-enough *love*.

Instead of love, I prefer to use the term *attunement*. Early experiences of attunement will, at a basic sensory level, engender *hope* and the sense that the world is a safe-enough place. This hope will be expressed in seeking therapy and, subsequently, in the willingness to accept what the therapist offers. Accordingly, for therapy to continue beyond the first few minutes of the meeting, the therapist must be able to offer themselves and their resources to the client in a way that resonates with this basic experience of hope.

What transpires in the first session can usually guide the ongoing process. By attending to the components outlined below, we can create a good-enough beginning in which the client feels seen and heard by the therapist and feels invited to return. The first session's main goal is to make the client want to come back.

Freud in his 1913 article *On Beginning the Treatment*, used the metaphor of a chess game to describe the nearly endless range of moves available to a skilled player. The same is true for the therapist. In the first moments of the initial session, all possibilities appear to be open. But, for the game to proceed, its rules must be followed, rules which are rigid. Freud's metaphor is limited in relation to the playfulness inherent in therapy, since in chess there is ultimately someone who wins and someone who loses. In therapy, the concept of winners and losers is irrelevant. Though the inherent power relations in the room need to be made apparent, winning or losing is not the goal. Freud's metaphor brings forth the crucial distinction between a *game*, based upon rigid rules and a victory at the end, and *playing*, based upon an imaginative and creative exchange with no apparent end in sight.

A more useful metaphor might be Winnicott's concepts of playfulness and the environmental mother, which refer to the pre-verbal aspects through which the dyadic relationship develops. These aspects help us understand the importance of the emotional environment and the role we, as therapists, play in its ongoing creation, establishment, and repair throughout the therapeutic hour.

The mother–infant unit is the most basic developmental unit of the individual. One cannot speak of the infant outside the context of this fundamental unit. When holding a baby, or an adult, we are taking care of the person. The individual is never alone. He is always a part of a holding environment, even if we are witnessing a severely damaged or lacking environment.

Such considerations are important when thinking about the environment we are creating for our work. There are physical and psychological aspects to such an environment in which we expect earlier patterns to be reenacted. When entering the room, the client will bring with them *traces* of his internalized environment to the environment we are providing.

The environment contains both verbal and nonverbal components, corresponding to conscious and unconscious elements. These distinctions do not represent a binary either–or perspective, but rather a both–and approach.

As can be inferred from the brief example at the start of the chapter, the emotional environment the therapist created outside the door was not optimal for Sue. It can be assumed that Sue will perceive the therapist as impatient, preoccupied with her own matters, and will therefore find it difficult to surrender to the process and to be open.

This initial meeting can be likened to the first meeting between a newborn baby and a mother exhausted from prolonged labour. The mother's desire for contact with her baby is not in question, but the experience she has just undergone makes it difficult for her to turn her attention away from her needs and towards the newborn. The same is true of the therapist Sue met.

Therapists working in the public sector, but not only there, often operate under physical and emotional conditions that make it difficult sometimes to establish the necessary environment to perform their work. Whether in a small office at social services, a therapy room in a boarding school, or a meeting room in a hospital, the existing conditions are often far from ideal. The room might be shared with other workers, making therapeutic dialogues difficult. The room might be in a noisy area, and its design or furnishings may be far from desirable. Nonetheless, even under less-than-optimal physical conditions, we must attempt to create the desired emotional environment. How should we go about doing that?

Being in the Room

The optimal physical space for therapy is a quiet room gently furnished and decorated and free from noisy design elements. The four walls of the room, including the windows and door, are the shape of the container, the holding experience, that every client seeks when coming to a first session.

It is a popular misconception that the room needs to be bare of any personal items that might attract the attention of the client and give away something about the subjectivity of the therapist. There is no reason to pretend that the therapist does not have a subjectivity. It will soon enough be reflected in the way they speak and respond to the client. Obviously, the room should not be cluttered in any way, reflecting the mind of the therapist, which is not cluttered by their own concerns but open to listening to and taking in the client. The therapist must arrange the room in such a way that feels comfortable and familiar for them to be spending the many hours they will in it, and at the same time leave enough room for the client. The client needs to feel that they can roam the room, mentally and physically, without feeling overwhelmed.

Attention should be paid to the seating arrangement in the room. In most public service offices, there are chairs, a desk, and sometimes armchairs. It is important to try to create at least one area where the therapist and client can sit without a desk between them. Sitting on opposite sides of a desk symbolizes too formal a relationship, which can hinder the openness necessary for therapy. Having said that, some clients might feel more comfortable with such a physical barrier, especially if the therapist is working for an agency that also has law-enforcement aspects to it.

Whether using chairs or armchairs, it is worth considering whether they face each other directly or are angled slightly. Armchairs placed directly opposite each other can create an overly intrusive experience in which the client has no choice but to look directly at the therapist. Armchairs positioned at a slight angle allow both the client and the therapist to look forward without necessarily making eye contact. This can create both a literal and symbolic space for gazing and internal reflection. This seating arrangement also symbolizes the uniqueness of the therapeutic session.

Generally, it is not recommended to sit beside the client, whether in chairs, armchairs, or even on a couch. Sitting side by side while facing the same direction has intimate social connotations and may convey an unintended message.

The room needs to be quiet to allow the voice of the client to be heard. The client needs to know that they are being listened to, both to the story they are telling aloud and to the inner one.

The client's voice, then, has two aspects: the external, conscious voice expressing their pain, and the inner, unconscious voice to which the therapist must also attune. The quietness shared by just the two of them in the room enables listening to both aspects. These are not in opposition; each tells a story, and the therapist must respond to both.

Of course, absolute quiet is not realistic. Every therapy room will suffer from some degree of background noise, which may distract or even pose a threat to the therapist's ability to listen and thus hinder the client's ability to express themselves. The same applies to seating arrangements, distractions, and physical accessibility. Any of these physical conditions may be lacking to some extent in the settings where therapeutic work takes place.

Whether they come due to marital difficulties, a mental health crisis, financial hardship, or any other reason, clients expect to meet in the figure of the therapist someone who can listen to and contain their experience. The room, therefore, is both a literal and symbolic representation of the containment the therapist offers simply by being willing to meet the person in distress.

Postponement of Satisfaction, or Wish Fulfilment?

> *Sue sits down across from Shelly and looks at her intently. Shelly lifts her head and is momentarily startled. Sitting in front of her is a fragile woman who looks frightened. She still feels shameful for having scolded her earlier. She smiles and asks Sue how she is.*
>
> *Sue asks if her brother can come in.*
>
> *Shelly hesitates.*

Shelly's dilemma whether to allow Sue's brother into the room, a request that might appear simple on the surface, touches upon one of the most enduring and basic questions in psychoanalytic psychotherapy: when a client articulates a wish or a need, should the good-enough therapist respond with gratification, recognizing the request as a developmentally appropriate expression of need? Or should the therapist withhold, understanding the request as a manifestation of unconscious fantasy or a reenactment of earlier repressed dynamics?

This question lies at the heart of a long-standing debate within psychoanalytic traditions. On the one hand, the view which evolved from schools of object relation theories acknowledges that, at times, the therapist must allow for a measure of satisfaction, even when this involves some deviation from strict therapeutic boundaries, lest the client retreat from therapy altogether. Here, concrete satisfaction of needs is seen as a precondition for building trust and for creating a holding environment that can support emotional growth.

On the other hand, the stricter position insists that gratification must be withheld so that the underlying unconscious conflicts, anxieties, and defences can surface. Only through the careful working through of frustration and transferential tension can the therapeutic relationship lead to enduring insight and structural change. Within this view, the therapist becomes less a caretaker and more an interpretive mirror, reflecting the client's internal world rather than immediately soothing it.

Sue arrives in acute distress at a space culturally and institutionally designated for care. Her presence is charged with emotional urgency, and her request carries with it the implicit cry of someone who has suffered a profound loss. Her appeal, framed as a need for her brother's presence, evokes the infant's call to the maternal figure: a plea for attunement, for immediate relief from mental pain. The urgency of this appeal naturally resonates within the therapist, potentially awakening countertransference responses rooted in guilt, anxiety, and the wish to repair.

Should Shelly respond in the spirit of the maternal caretaker and meet Sue's need without delay? Or should she pause, reflect, and consider the symbolic weight of the request, its manifest content and its latent emotional significance? This tension is not merely theoretical; it lives in the room, in Shelly's body and in her ethical deliberations.

The answer might appear simple and based on rational thought: clearly, Shelly should concretely grant Sue's request. Shelly also wonders whether Sue's request for her brother's presence represents a disruption of the emerging therapeutic dyad or a reparative gesture, an attempt to mend the disruption caused by Shelly's earlier, less attuned response. Shelly finds herself cast in the role of the mother who feels the pain of having failed her infant and now seeks to repair. But does repair in this moment mean total gratification? Or might it mean holding the boundary and allowing the meaning of that earlier empathic failure to slowly reveal itself?

Such clinical moments resist easy answers. They call for the therapist's capacity to hold ambiguity, to dwell in the space between action and reflection. The ethical and clinical task, then, is not simply to gratify or to frustrate, but to listen deeply to what is said and what is enacted, and to respond in a way that preserves the integrity of the therapeutic frame while remaining open to its transformation. Several factors need to be considered.

Shelly needs to consider the cultural difference. What does the presence of another person –Sue's brother or even an interpreter – mean within Sue's cultural background? Could the presence of her brother, a man, prevent Sue from truly expressing the distress she might hope to share with another woman? Perhaps Sue is asking for her brother's presence in order to appease him, or the authorities, while in fact his presence might impede her openness? There are many ways of looking at this, and it might only be in hindsight that the "correct" option becomes clear. I suggest that what is most significant is to try and consider all options in order to facilitate the best conditions possible. But still be ready for a surprise without feeling too guilty about making the "wrong" choice.

She would also be advised to consider whether their less-than-ideal first impression echoes a personal experience of Sue's. If so, should Shelly compensate for this impression by complying with Sue's request to have her brother present?

Therefore, even before the first session properly begins, the therapist is already dealing with profound questions that help shape their position towards the client. Conscious decisions need to be made while paying close attention to unconscious complications. It is never a matter of saying yes or no to the client.

The Therapeutic Contract and Alliance

> *Shelly proposes to Sue that the two of them first meet without the brother or the interpreter, who is waiting in the adjoining room, and conduct the conversation in English. Sue agrees. Shelly explains to Sue that everything she shares will remain confidential, unless there is a risk to her life or she is aware of an imminent criminal act. She then asks Sue why she has come to see her.*

Shelly's decision reveals that she has made a clinical decision based upon ethical considerations. Regarding *confidentiality*, she decided that this is a basic condition. Although it frustrates the client's request, Shelly views maintaining confidentiality as essential. Despite the apparent clash between the client's request and the formal framework, Shelly made her decision based on ethical and professional principles: maintaining formal confidentiality is key to allowing the epistemic trust required for therapy.

Part of Shelly's rationale also relates to *cultural sensitivity*. She understands that while Sue might feel more comfortable with someone from her own culture present as an interpreter so that she can use her mother tongue, the potential frustration about this absence is less critical than the risk that another person's presence would inhibit Sue's freedom in saying what is really troubling her.

Shelly also considered the interaction that already took place between her and Sue. She decided that even though she feels guilty for not responding to Sue's initial need, she acted for reasons not yet fully understood. She should not try to compensate concretely for that guilt. Shelly assumes that this *empathic failure* will turn out to be meaningful both in the *transference* that will develop between them and as part of Sue's reason for seeking therapy in the first place.

Each of these aspects leads Shelly to make a formal decision that essentially marks the first stage in establishing *the therapeutic contract and alliance*.

The therapeutic *contract* and the therapeutic *alliance* describe the conscious agreement, *contract*, made between therapist and client which allows for the safe containment, *alliance*, of the unconscious elements.

The therapeutic contract is the formal aspect of the relationship, as I have specified earlier, and relates to time management etc. Once these elements are agreed upon, the emotional foundation of the relationship is established, allowing for the alliance to emerge based upon trust, attunement, and hope. Inevitably, there will be discrepancies between the two frames as unconscious material begins to seep through and influence the formal aspects of the relationship through the workings of *transference* and *repetition compulsion*. This is the stuff that therapy is made of, and here the work begins.

For example, Shelly offered Sue a contract that included confidentiality and exclusivity, especially the exclusion of any third party from their conversations. This is a concrete and conscious element, yet it enables the unconscious experience of *epistemic trust* between them, which is a key component of the therapeutic alliance. It creates a space where Shelly's full attention is focused solely on Sue's subjective experience, free from external influences.

In a sense, by trusting Shelly and accepting the terms of the contract, Sue allows a certain suspension of her autonomy. This suspension also reflects the non-reciprocal nature of the therapeutic relationship. She sees the therapist as a professional authority and entrusts herself to their care. This trust forms the basis of the therapeutic *contract*, thereby enabling the therapeutic *alliance*.

Free Association, Free Listening

Sue looks shyly at Shelly; she tries to relax, telling herself that she might be able to trust Shelly, eventually. Something about Shelly's smile now seems reassuring. Sue can hear voices in the hallway and hopes her own words won't be overheard. She begins to share her story. She went through the long and expensive process of migration in her homeland and says, with hesitance, that she wanted to get away from the Philippines for several reasons, and Shelly can see she is not yet ready to expand on this. The work she has found in Israel as a carer for elderly people is relatively good. The woman Sue is looking after is kind, but nights have been tough as the woman wakes up regularly.

Shelly listens with genuine interest. The language and cultural gaps seem irrelevant. As a social worker in Tel Aviv, Shelly is familiar with such stories. Technically, the welfare office may not be the ideal place for Sue's case, and Shelly wonders how she can help.

Sue pauses mid-sentence, seemingly deciding what to say next. Shelly could encourage her to stay on topic or leave space for something unexpected and revealing to emerge.

Even in the first moments of an initial meeting, before the reason for the referral is fully clear, the therapist needs to just listen to whatever the client chooses to say, as I have expanded upon in the Chapter One. Such listening to the client's free associations is focused not only on what is being said but also on how it is said. Shelly allowed herself to be influenced emotionally by both the content and tone of the narrative.

There is of course no such thing as purely free association. When we speak, there is always a connection between the things we say. Mostly, with most people, the connection is rational and makes sense, but sometimes it may indeed be unconscious, and that is where the notion of free becomes more apparent. It is free in the sense that it is not constrained or directed by what we aim to understand. We listen with as open a mind as possible, knowing that some of the connections will only be made eventually, through our insight into the underlying unconscious layer of the self.

There is another very important and inevitable complication here. The freedom with which the speech of the client moves forward is also consciously and unconsciously determined by what they sense is allowed by our free listening. So, the freedom of associations and listening is more a goal that we forever strive towards rather than a technical description of what takes place.

Becoming increasingly aware of the constraints of the client's associations and our listening allows us to understand what earlier patterns are being repeated in the transference. These constraints are slowly understood as the client's and our own defence mechanisms, repeated in the unique unfolding relationship we form with the client.

A further complication arises in this particular case as Sue is not able to express herself freely in a language which is not her mother tongue. Such an instance is quite common today as immigration has become so common in so many countries. In Israel alone there are at least a dozen different languages used by different communities, and no one therapist can be expected to be fluent in all of them. Most Israeli therapists whose Hebrew or Arabic is their mother tongue speak good-enough English to be able to conduct an adequate therapeutic dialogue. It is far from perfect and often the presence of an interpreter is required, thus complicating questions of confidentiality as shown earlier.

When a safe-enough space is created, clients often say things they hadn't initially intended. These new revelations may not be secrets, but they often reflect deeper issues which have led the client to seek help. Sue may have approached Shelly with one issue, but once she felt secure, other, more pressing concerns surfaced.

Listening to these hidden or semi-hidden contents is a hallmark of psychoanalytic psychotherapy. The goal isn't simply to expose secrets but to help clients better understand themselves and thereby use their internal resources to improve their condition.

What Sue shared when she felt safe enough, after about halfway through the session, wasn't unconscious content; she had been actively hiding it until she felt ready. In the early stages of therapy, the unconscious aspects of the therapist–client relationship remain largely unexamined. Even though the underlying unconscious processes are already at work, the therapist must be careful not to make early assumptions about their meaning and interpret them too soon. It can take weeks, months, and maybe longer before the therapist can be certain enough of having a firm grasp as to the role they are playing unconsciously in the unfolding narrative. Therefore, it is best to wait rather than speak too soon and take the risk of appearing to be intrusive and presumptuous.

Making an interpretation too early, before the client is ready to hear it, might lead to a breach in the alliance. If that happens, it does not mean that it is irreversible and damaging. In most cases it will signify another important unconscious process that has been going on that needs to be addressed. The breach can be mended and thus reinforce the alliance. The ability of the good-enough therapist to acknowledge their own failings is an important aspect of the therapeutic process. This does not necessarily mean that the therapist needs to apologize for errors made, though that is quite alright to do, but rather to try and understand their mistakes in the wider context of the transference and unconscious communication. As I will expand on in other chapters, such errors are best considered not just as ordinary and human mistakes made by the therapist but as potentially the result of *projective identification*, whereby unwanted parts of the client are projected onto the therapist, enabling, or forcing them, to act upon them.

To Focus or Not to Focus? That is the Question: Towards the End of the First Session

> *After a minute or two of silence, Sue says to Shelly that she has something she wants to share, something that has been troubling her for a long time. She tells her that the person accompanying her and sitting outside in the corridor is not actually her brother but her husband.*
>
> *He arrived in Israel before her. They had decided to present themselves as siblings because they believed it would be easier to find work that way. They had*

heard that if they were discovered to be a married couple they would be immediately deported due to official Israeli policies. For the most part, they had managed to conceal the nature of their relationship, but recently they had begun to worry because one of their acquaintances had discovered the truth and was threatening to report them to the immigration authorities. Additionally, they had come to the decision that they wanted children but were afraid of the implications of such a step.

When a client unexpectedly discloses some piece of information or a significant experience near the end of a first session, the therapist might assume that the alliance formed is strong enough, or that the crisis is harsher than realized.

These are two very different possible courses of clinical action. If the client disclosed due to feeling safe enough, that is a good sign that the process is going well, and the therapist can acknowledge the disclosure and reassure the client that they will help them deal with the situation in later sessions. However, if the disclosure is a result of an acute state of distress, the therapist needs to consider a possible line of action beyond the scope of the therapeutic hour.

Either way, it seems that Sue presented an issue that can be conceptualized as *the central problem*. This central problem, or symptom, may serve as the guiding signpost for the therapy. Naturally, the therapeutic process will open up additional dimensions, but this initial, basic experience forms the primary layer of the therapeutic relationship, in a way reminiscent of an infant's first year of life.

Just as the first minutes of the first session are important and may serve as a microcosm of the entire process, special attention should also be paid to how the first session approaches its end. In the final minutes of the session, the therapist should share with the client both their initial professional impressions regarding the therapeutic potential and the basic rules that form the therapeutic contract.

It is important that the client leaves the session equipped with meaningful information regarding both aspects – content and framework. If the client chooses to continue, they must consciously understand and accept the formal therapeutic framework, and yet, for this space to feel subjectively meaningful to them, they must experience a certain intimacy that makes them feel like they will want to return for future sessions.

Sue gets up from her seat and makes for the corridor where her husband is waiting. He looks worried. She lingers for a moment in the doorway to smile back at Shelly, who has walked her to the door and now reminds Sue what time their next appointment is.

Starting and ending therapy is more than simply showing up at a set time in a set place. It is a meaningful turning point, a fragile meeting between two strangers who are learning how to move between distance and closeness. Just as a newborn's first breath carries the whole promise of life, the first moments of a session hold within them the potential of everything that might follow.

In stepping hesitantly across Shelly's doorway, Sue shows the great courage it takes to place one's pain in another person's hands. Her glance back at her husband, back at the familiar, reflects the central tension of therapy: the pull between safety and risk, between hiding and opening up.

The beginning of therapy is never perfect or fully predictable. It always carries traces of past relationships. It is in these very imperfections, Shelly's brief sharpness, Sue's guarded story, that the real work begins. The therapist's ability to stay attentive not only to what is said but also to what is left unsaid is what allows trust to take root.

Hope in therapy does not rest on promises of a cure. It rests instead on the therapist's deep belief in people's ability to change through words and connection. This hope, born of both skill and compassion, creates the invisible container that allows the client to risk being vulnerable.

Chapter 4

The Supervisory Quartet

How Institutional Containment Transforms Psychoanalytic Supervision in Multicultural Settings

The significance of supervision in therapeutic professions extends far beyond routine professional requirements. It is the stage upon which the phenomenon of *transference*, which I see as central to psychotherapy, can be played out and observed. Without consistent and attuned supervisory presence, the therapist risks becoming trapped in repetitive patterns with the client that perpetuate rather than resolve difficulties.

Supervision is one of the cornerstones of psychoanalytic training. As such, it allows the therapist to examine the intricate dynamics of the therapeutic relationship. Beyond the consideration of the client's presenting symptoms and the possible ways of understanding them, it investigates the deeper emotional undercurrents that flow beneath conscious awareness.

The Structure of Supervisory Practice

Supervision exists as an inherently triangular structure, involving supervisor, supervisee, and client in a complex configuration that requires careful containment. This three-way dynamic often mirrors certain aspects of early dynamics of all three participants.

Supervision also operates within a hierarchical structure not unlike other apprenticeship systems, where expertise is transmitted through careful mentorship. In this model, the material brought to supervision becomes raw material to be refined through the supervisor's greater clinical experience and theoretical knowledge. The supervisor's role resembles that of a master craftsperson, helping the supervisee identify and address the inevitable blind spots that obscure even well-intentioned therapeutic work.

But supervision is seldom straightforward or simple because the unconscious processes of both supervisor and supervisee inevitably weave themselves into the relationship's matrix. These unconscious forces inevitably shape, and occasionally enact, dynamics that reach far deeper than conscious awareness or intention.

Some supervision relationships focus primarily on symptom management and case coordination, thereby avoiding these deeper psychological territories.

DOI: 10.4324/9781003683162-4

These approaches reflect the practical realities of contemporary mental health systems. The declining resources available to public-sector mental health and social work services create pressures that favour rapid intervention over in-depth exploration.

Regardless of the kind of approach therapists use, they need to be in supervision, especially during the early stages of their career. It can be argued that once the therapist has accumulated many hours of supervision, that figure becomes internalized and acts as an *internal supervisor* or *observing self*, adjacent to his *superego*. Nevertheless, as the mind never rests, it is essential to continue looking into the flexibility and authenticity of that internal supervisor's capacity and to highlight unconscious dimensions, which will always be there. Even when the therapist is very experienced and supervises other younger therapists, the unconscious undercurrents will never cease to activate areas in their experience that need to be looked at. I suggest that these undercurrents can be seen as *parallel processes* that are evoked by material brought up by the client and need to be looked at carefully so that the therapist themselves, and the supervisor in turn, don't act upon them.

The concept of parallel process captures for me one of supervision's most intriguing and challenging aspects, the remarkable correspondence between the supervisee's experiences in supervision and the client's experiences in therapy. This mirroring effect operates like an endless series of reflections, each containing and reflecting the others in a continuous cycle of psychological projection and identification.

When parallel processes are not considered and looked at, supervision work may stall. In such a case, the power of *repetition compulsion* emerges to reenact the client's unresolved conflicts within supervision itself. The supervisee, unknowingly, assumes the client's position, while the supervisor steps into the therapeutic role, thus repeating rather than resolving the issues at hand.

The supervisor's tendency to identify with the supervisee's internalized relationship patterns creates a complex interplay with the client's parallel tendency to identify with the supervisee's internal world. This intricate psychological matrix, while present in all supervisory relationships, becomes increasingly difficult to recognize, understand, and skilfully manage when therapy ventures into areas of *primitive emotional development*.

The realm of primitive emotional development reveals how the earliest developmental injuries create transference dynamics of extraordinary complexity and intensity. These early wounds, like fault lines in psychological development, generate reverberations that continue throughout the individual's life.

Clients who have experienced early developmental injuries, regardless of their specific nature, often develop *defence mechanisms* of considerable toxicity, as I have explored in previous chapters. These defences manifest in the *transference* through *acting out* rather than words. The client uses actions to repeat and express their deepest pain, requiring the therapist to serve as a container for experiences that resist verbal articulation.

In such cases, the supervisee inevitably carries the impact of these intense sessions into the supervision space, where these elements risk being *acted out* again rather than processed and understood. Supervision becomes a potential stage for repeating the client's most primitive communications, requiring special attention and awareness to transform *acting out* into *insight*. In fact, in such cases, you could say that the supervisors themselves need to be supervised. This can take place either through an additional layer of supervision, or, as I will demonstrate later, through the special case of the presence of the agency in which therapy takes place.

Psychotherapy Within a Hierarchical Institution

Supervision inherently contains an educational component, which needs to be watched so it does not overwhelm the relationship's therapeutic potential. The traditional educational model positions the supervisor as teacher and guide, with interactions focused primarily on one-way knowledge transmission from experienced professional to developing practitioner. This emphasis on supervisory authority, while offering obvious benefits, can rigidify into an overly hierarchical structure that constrains the free-floating attention and associative processes essential to psychoanalytic work. Such rigidity may infantilize the supervisee, positioning them as helplessly dependent rather than as an active participant in a collaborative exploration of unconscious processes.

A more productive perspective views the supervisor as an equal contributor within the supervisory triangle, not equal in experience or knowledge, but equal in their capacity of being under the same influence of unconscious patterns. This approach might be criticized for potentially blurring the essential distinction between therapy and supervision, risking the development of professional awareness into personal treatment. It might neglect the ethical dimensions crucial to professional learning, creating a space where the supervisor merely addresses the supervisee's emotional distress rather than guiding their work professionally.

I propose, however, that therapy and supervision are siblings in the psychoanalytic process, sharing common borders while maintaining separate identities. Both positions adhere to the same ethical standards and engage in deep exploration of unconscious processes, yet they differ fundamentally in their primary focus and ultimate objectives.

In personal therapy, the individual's journey begins with their own material. In supervision, the supervisee initially addresses the client's concerns, yet the exploration may naturally expand to include the supervisee's own responses without losing sight of the ultimate goal: helping the client with their own process.

No therapeutic work occurs in isolation; every therapist practises within a specific framework, whether a private clinic's setting, a social services agency's bureaucratic complexity, or a special needs school. The agency's context creates a unique frame that influences both therapeutic and supervisory processes.

The agency's presence – its objectives, policies, and cultural norms – adds another layer to the client–supervisee–supervisor triangle. These institutional forces operate both explicitly and implicitly, consciously and unconsciously, weaving themselves into the fabric of therapeutic and supervisory relationships like an invisible *fourth participant* whose influence must be acknowledged.

An example of this is the code for ethical conduct regarding sexual boundaries. An agency will have such a code not merely as bureaucratic regulation but as a framework that protects both client vulnerability and therapist professional integrity. When a member of the therapeutic triad – therapist, supervisor, or client – behaves in ways that violate institutional codes, the agency itself becomes an active participant in the matrix. The once-triangular structure of supervision suddenly expands into *a four-way configuration*, a quartet, with institutional authority stepping forward as a visible participant rather than remaining in the background as an invisible influence.

The following fictional case study will illustrate some of these points. It is based upon my own experience as a supervisor in various social work settings in Israel as well as upon my experience as a university lecturer.

Cutural Codes

Mike was a Christian Arab male in his mid-twenties, a third and final year student doing his BA in Social Work, which I supervised around the year 2001 while he was on placement in a special-needs primary school in Jaffa, a mixed Arab-Jewish city in Israel, where he practised play therapy with children.

He was doing well in his placement, after some initial difficulty, and the staff of the school, including the counsellor and the educational psychologist, were pleased both with his reports of play therapy and with his consultations with them. He seemed to be reasonably enjoying his placement, though at times he seemed to be downcast and was preoccupied with something he did not share. Was it an impasse, I wondered, or was it a matter of him gaining more confidence in his work and needing more reassurance and containment before he could dare to be more open?

Sometime after the placement was underway, he arrived in school wearing a sleeveless shirt, which was unusual in relation to how all other men dressed in that school. I noticed it straight away and felt puzzled by it. At first, I was not sure if I had to do something about it, even though it was commented upon by other staff members as being perhaps an inappropriate way for a student to dress. I did not say anything during or after that first time, but when he continued to appear at school wearing the same or very similar top, I discussed it with a female colleague, who thought that no boundaries were crossed and advised me to wait it out.

A couple of weeks later, the director of the local Social Services department visited the school and was introduced to the school's staff. The visit itself proceeded well, but a couple of days later I received a phone call from her. The director approached the subject of what was and what was not appropriate as a dress code in the school. She asked me to consider the possibility that Mike's choice of dress was perhaps a statement, perhaps partially unconscious, either regarding the placement, or regarding the supervision. She asked me to consider what course of action I wanted to take. It was clear that I could not just continue to deny it.

Personal vs.Political

I found myself considering her remark within two different but related fields. It was an intersubjective issue within the supervision, touching upon *authority* within *transference*. It also concerned cultural assumptions and power. In other words, was the dilemma a clinical one, resulting from an incident of acting-out within the supervision transference, or a political one, resulting from gender and national and cultural issues? With time I came to see that it was both.

Jaffa is one of the oldest cities in the world, even mentioned in the Old Testament. After the establishment of Israel, it was incorporated into Tel Aviv, the country's largest city. Today, most of its residents are Muslim and Christian Arabs, all citizens of Israel. A Jewish minority has lived in Jaffa for centuries, and in recent decades their numbers and influence have grown as more Jews moved in, bought houses, and contributed to the city's development, a process some call "gentrification".

Jaffa itself is indeed a mixed city and represents often the pluralistic and liberal nature that most Israelis aspire to. Jewish and Arab families often live in the same neighbourhoods, sometimes even in the same buildings. In recent years, the mix has grown more diverse with the arrival of African immigrants and refugees, many of whom lack residence permits and settle in the inner-city areas.

Ever since Jewish immigration resumed in the 19th century after two millennia of exile, Israel has wrestled with questions of identity, coexistence, and racism, both individual and institutional. The repeated wars with Arab neighbours and with Palestinians in the West Bank and Gaza have left their mark. In mixed cities like Jaffa, the friction is often palpable, but alongside the tension there is also genuine coexistence: not only as a slogan but as a warm, lively, and optimistic reality.

The school where I worked was a secular, liberal primary school that respected all three religions, Muslim, Christian, and Jewish. Both pupils and staff came from varied cultural and religious backgrounds. While the school was part of Tel Aviv's mainstream education system, over time it became a place where children with behavioural and emotional challenges were referred. Many were diagnosed with conditions such as ADHD, Oppositional Defiant Disorder, or Conduct Disorder.

Most pupils came from low socioeconomic backgrounds and from different cultural, ethnic, and national communities. Some lived in foster families, others in residential homes after being removed from their parents' care because of neglect or abuse. The staff was just as diverse, including not only teachers but also therapists from different disciplines. They offered individual and group therapy, from weekly sessions to daily group meetings. The teaching and therapy teams met regularly to consult, review progress, and ensure that interventions were effective.

As I reflected on these issues, I was aware of the complexities of my position as a Jewish member of the majority group in Israel, especially when holding a role of relative authority in a supervisory setting. My own sense of ease in addressing national and cultural differences may be connected to this majority position, while for Mike, my supervisee, the experience could be different.

The Impasse

I began thinking of the *impasse* as a *symptom*. Therefore, I went back in my mind and tried to see if there was something that I should have noticed in the early stages of the placement and the supervision. I was also aware that that kind of thinking implied that I was thinking of Mike as a client and not as just a supervisee.

The supervision was going relatively well, but I recalled and read in my notes that it did not start like that. Mike's initial request for this placement was to work with adults in a mental health setting. Due to various circumstances, this was not possible, and he was placed in the school. When I first met him, he complained about this and was very resentful towards the university for not granting his request.

We spoke quite a lot during the first supervision session about the real professional challenges he was facing. It was becoming clearer that some of his objections to the placement in that school were to do with his lack of confidence in his ability to work well with children. Regarding academic requirements and previous experience, he did have sufficient ability for the placement. He was meant to undertake at least one course of play therapy as well as participating in group activities and staff meetings.

I did have my residual doubts as to whether it was always safe and wise to let young students work with children who were often very hurt children. When Mike expressed his displeasure at even being there, I had to be careful and listen to him and not let my own bias overshadow the situation at hand. My assessment at the time was that as a student he should be able to adjust himself to the situation and accept the placement as it was. I conveyed that to him clearly but was also empathic with his difficulty.

During the following weeks, after the induction period was over and Mike became more familiar with the setting of the school, he began to fulfil his assignments. He did this well, and I found myself even surprised as to how quickly he had adjusted himself, considering how upset he was previously.

Focusing on the easier overt option that dealing with the dress code offered me, I had to check with the school's administration whether such a dress code indeed existed. I soon discovered that there was no written school rule detailing the acceptable dress code for adults. Of course, pupils were expected to dress according to written rules which were both explicit and printed out on the wall in various places throughout the school.

As there were no written rules for adults, I had to ask myself whether Mike's code of dress interfered with his professional behaviour in general, and particularly working with children at the school. It was not enough to pass a judgement upon his dress as such (the action itself) but to consider the maxim of the action (the action in context). I wanted to be on firm ground on this and not be led astray by my own bias.

The question of authority in a supervision relationship between an Israeli Jew and an Arab Christian is a political issue. Being part of a minority placed Mike in a subjectively more vulnerable position. I could not rule out the possibility that he felt unsafe in the school due to that. It was possible that he was keeping his real political sentiments to himself. Was his dress a signifier of a deeper sentiment he dared not express openly? I had seen him talking and behaving seemingly freely and openly with other colleagues, both Jews and Arabs, and got the impression that he felt at ease in the liberal atmosphere of the school. Could it be that Mike was *acting out* in the *transference*? If so, what was being acted out rather than remembered?

When I brought up the issue during our next session, we were able to work through this carefully. I suggested to Mike that his dress was indicative of a thought or a feeling that perhaps he was not fully aware of and suggested that we talk about this. Luckily, after his initial embarrassment, he welcomed this intervention. I was relieved that he did not feel too admonished, even though I did share with him that it was the Social Services director's intervention that made me realize something was not being discussed. What follows is the narrative we both were able to piece together during the following sessions, which led to the good-enough resolution of the impasse.

> *Mike had found himself in a placement he did not want to be in. His wish for a specific placement was frustrated by the decision taken by the university. He felt powerless and hard done by. He felt that his genuine interest and ability went unrecognized and even ignored by the agency and the university. Nevertheless, his actual experience during the first few days at the school was fulfilling. He found himself enjoying what he was learning. Still, he had a lingering feeling that it could have been better.*
>
> *He said that when he first met me he was impressed by my welcoming smile. He soon learnt to acknowledge our work together as beneficial and found the sessions very helpful. More than that, he even liked me, a little bit more than he had allowed himself to admit. To his friends, he spoke of a good-looking Jewish therapist who was very knowledgeable. He masked his own interest by suggested to his friends that he thought I was also gay and fancied him, even though I showed no sign of it. He felt embarrassed by it but also not able to ignore his sensations. He knew what transference-love was; he had studied it and felt awkward about it.*

Since Freud's 1915 paper *Observations on Transference-Love*, the phenomenon of transference-love has remained one of psychoanalysis's most challenging clinical issues. Despite Freud's acknowledgement that discussion of this topic was already overdue in 1915, relatively little was written about transference-love until the 1990s, when several intersubjective and relational psychoanalytic theorists, including Lewis Aron (1952–2019), Glen Gabbard (b. 1949), and Christopher Bollas, began exploring the subject with renewed theoretical rigor and clinical candour.

While the scope of this book cannot adequately address the full complexity of *transference-love*, it is possible to outline two predominant theoretical perspectives. The first view conceptualizes the emergence of transference-love as a manifestation of *resistance*, arising when the client experiences an imminent threat of exposing repressed material, typically related to early sexual conflicts and oedipal dynamics. According to this classical approach, the therapist should interpret and work through the resistance as they would any other defensive manoeuvre, thereby allowing the therapeutic process to continue without obstruction.

The second perspective, representing a more contemporary and nuanced understanding, views transference-love as an almost inevitable occurrence within intensive therapeutic relationships. This approach conceptualizes such feelings as an expression of *affectionate transference* that facilitates access to deeper layers of emotional development. From this point of view, the careful exploration of transference-love, rather than its immediate interpretation as resistance, can lead to significant therapeutic breakthroughs, enabling clients to develop greater psychological freedom in expressing and fulfilling their capacity for mature adult relationships.

Central to this second approach is the principle that exploring transference-love within appropriate therapeutic boundaries allows clients to remember and work through repressed aspects of early relationships rather than enacting them through boundary violations or other forms of acting out. Without such awareness, the appearance of transference-love can often lead to an impasse in the process. Both client and therapist are locked together in a situation they are not fully aware of. Such a situation becomes threatening so that an impasse seems like a logical defence mechanism. It is better to stay still and frozen in an impasse rather than move forward deeper into contacting unresolved, possibly painful memories and experiences. If an impasse results from unconscious reenactment rather than conscious remembering, it becomes crucial to understand what underlying dynamics are being acted out rather than therapeutically processed.

The Quartet of Transference

Having explored Mike's contribution to this dynamic, our investigation turned towards examining the client with whom he was working and the specific transference matrix that emerged between them. He was working with an 11-year-old Muslim girl, Basmat, who lived with foster parents after having been removed from her parents' care after being sexually abused by her stepfather five years earlier, when she was 6 years old. Basmat's mother suffered from chronic schizophrenia and as she was often in hospital was found to be unable to care for her daughter . The abuse involved the stepfather exposing the girl to pornographic materials on the internet and suggesting to her that he showed her "how it was being done". Basmat told her previous schoolteacher about his suggestions, and social services intervened, finding a household on the brink of collapse. Basmat was removed from her parents' care and placed with a foster home.

Basmat had been in intensive therapy in previous years, and Mike's goal in meeting her was to help her further develop her social skills. It had been noticed that she tended to be over-dominant with her friends. Mike found Basmat to be a likeable and talkative girl and formed a warm connection with her very quickly.

Nevertheless, knowing she had been abused was intimidating. Working on his session reports in our supervision sessions, we were forming the opinion that Basmat was presenting overdominance in her interactions with her peers as a reaction formation regarding her fear of being abused again.

During that time, Mike had a frightening dream from which he awoke with a start. The dream showed a young boy being chased down a long corridor by male figures who seemed to want to drag him into a box. In the following session, he told me the dream. I had instructed him to monitor closely his dreams, as they had the potential to shed light upon the unconscious communication between him and Basmat. Mike shared that dream in supervision with some reluctance, as he was ashamed of it.

He felt it was too revealing. He rationalized that as a way of maintaining his sense of autonomy in the supervision. It was then he began arriving at school wearing a sleeveless shirt.

Mike's dress choice was an instance of acting-out within supervision. Until it was worked through, Mike's repressed ambivalence was expressed by his sleeveless shirt. It allowed him a peek at violating boundaries, a repetition of content that seeped through from his therapy and activated a part of him he dared not express openly.

Basmat has suffered sexual injury, which was only partially and indirectly brought up in her play during her therapy sessions. Mike had formed a good therapeutic alliance with Basmat and felt attuned to her. That meant he was also receptive to unconscious communication. When discussing his dream, he could see that it contained a reference to a projected part of Basmat's undigested injured mind.

Mike's unconscious identification with that projected part indicated the good rapport he had established with her. The dream represented an expression of that projection and remained an undigested and painful mental item.

In a sense, it was only in that way that Mike was able to represent his tension in the supervision, tension which had been building up since the beginning of the placement.

In my own therapy during that time, I was able to work through my part. I realized I was overcompensating for my discomfort regarding Mike's disappointment. I was going out of my way to try and accommodate his request for changes in the times of our meeting, allowed him to be absent from staff meetings without properly exploring it, and generally treated him as if he himself was an injured child. It was that special treatment which left room for Mike to develop that transference-love rather than give full and direct expression to his angst. He substituted his anger with love, which I had allowed by relaxing the boundaries.

The agency's role, the fourth player in this quartet of transference, was in a sense the container of the whole situation. It is the kind of containment which I argue is always present in the therapy room, even if that room is in a private clinic, where no one sees what is going on. It is most often represented by the ethical code each therapist must abide by, regardless of whether they are social workers, psychologist, psychiatrist, clinical criminologist, or any other professional working in such a capacity. Mostly, such containment is silent and can easily be seen as being held by the mind of the therapist.

It is in cases such as severe abuse occurring early in childhood that that internal good-enough parent object is damaged and starts to malfunction. Its absence, or partial absence, then sends ripples through the therapeutic dyad and the supervisory triangle, showing up as threats to the safe boundaries of the therapy. Those ripples can cause acting out in the behaviour of each of the participants in the quartet. Without any of those participants becoming aware of these ripples and their threatening nature, therapeutic and supervisory relationships can go wrong. In some cases when they go very wrong, we read about them in the paper. We know that boundary crossing in psychotherapy is under-reported and that there are many clients, therapists, and supervisors out there who have gone astray.

All these insights were discussed and worked through during the following supervision sessions, as well as in a meeting I held with the Social Services director. Despite the initial embarrassment that was experienced both by Mike and me, we were eventually able to marvel together at the wonders of the unconscious. The placement continued, as did Mike's work with Basmat. During the supervision sessions, we were able to use the insights gained to further develop our understanding of the triadic situation in its complexity.

The traditional aim of supervision is for the supervisor to support the supervisee in their work with the client, so that *transference* and *resistance* are dealt with in such a way that all parties benefit from it, and especially the client. As I have argued, it is by no means a single directional process and must be looked at as a system. The role of the fourth, silent partner must also be considered.

The involvement of an agency in supervision, turning the triad into a quartet, can be inhibitory but also beneficial. It is my opinion that the agency, or the ethical code, as was shown in this case, can facilitate a better understanding of the supervision practice and illuminate unconscious aspects. That insight is vital for learning, which is and must always be the driving force in supervision and therapy.

Chapter 5

The Contained and the Container

Erotic Transference as Annihilation in Psychoanalytic Psychotherapy

In this chapter, I will describe yet another instance of transference, as I see transference as the main arena where psychoanalytic psychotherapy takes place. I describe a different class of *transference-love, erotic transference*, which disrupts the therapeutic alliance beyond repair. Transference-love and erotic transference are closely related but not the same. In transference-love, a client feels strong affection, admiration, or idealization towards the therapist. These feelings often echo early childhood relationships and unmet needs for care, attention, or validation. In erotic transference, the feelings include sexual attraction or fantasies directed towards the therapist. Both forms involve the client unconsciously repeating past patterns in therapy. The similarity is that both reflect deep emotional needs being re-experienced in the present. The difference is that erotic transference carries a distinctly and often active sexual tone, while transference-love may remain non-sexual. I will show what can happen in cases when the therapeutic alliance, comes under an attack through erotic transference that is too great for it to sustain.

Therapeutic Alliance

Therapeutic alliance refers to the client's willingness to accept the therapist's aid in overcoming their difficulties. It includes their acceptance of the need to deal with their pain and accept the boundaries of therapeutic work, even when faced with resistance.

When this alliance comes under attack, especially in the guise of erotic transference as this chapter will explore, the ongoing treatment is threatened. Once unconscious materials are getting nearer the surface, they become threatening to the emotional status quo the client has reached in their life, even if that state is a pathological one.

This is the work of *transference*, triggering early patterns that the individual has struggled to guard against. Therapy becomes an arena where the past becomes too real and forgotten and denied events become alive, exposing the client to what seems like real danger.

DOI: 10.4324/9781003683162-5

When transference enters the realm of love in a disruptive fashion, the matrix of the therapy is under pressure, jeopardizing the introspective and reflective subjective processes. It seems that sometimes the mind prefers to get worse rather than risk change. Ultimately, this might turn into the worst, suicide.

There are two opposing forces at work here. The first one is the ambivalent connection with the therapist, driven by an unconscious repetition of an unresolved conflict or an enactment of an early relational pattern. This force is often destructive, seeking to repeat what is already familiar, though painful. The second force is represented by the client's rational resolve to be an active partner in the therapeutic relationship aimed at bringing about internal change.

The conflict between these two forces is often staged within *the therapeutic setting*. A threat to the setting need not always be a problem. It can even be a creative expression of the client's growing autonomy. In the process of seeking new experiences, the client may well playfully ask questions regarding what seems to be obvious. Issues of time, payment, frequency of sessions, and the therapist's privacy are good issues to be discussed. This can be a sign of health. The client is renewing their strength or gaining access to it for the first time. They might feel equal to the therapist and challenge them as part of a good-enough *Oedipal process*. If the playful nature of such a challenge is contained and the therapy continues, there is no threat to the alliance.

It is when such challenges becomes toxic and subverted into *acting-out* that the *alliance* is in danger, requiring the therapist to continuously repair and sustain it. In his book *The Dove that Returns, The Dove that Vanishes,* Michael Parsons (b. 1941) likens this repairing and maintenance of the setting to the work of the farmer who mends his fences after the storm, knowing he will have to do so again as part of his work.

The therapist will do the same with care, bearing in mind that any attacks upon the setting could be expressions of the client's vitality and engagement with the process. The client, who is asking for help as a result of damage sustained to their primitive relationship with others, is bound to act out very difficult scenes in the setting of the therapy room before a positive change can take place. These scenes may well be expressions of sheer hatred towards the therapist and must be contained for the journey to progress. The therapist needs to survive those attacks.

The story I will now share with you is of such dimensions. Sadly, I could not fully contain the storms that erupted in the room. It was indeed a tale of erotic transference turned into devastating hatred.

Hatred in the Room

The tale is of Amanda, a client diagnosed with *borderline personality disorder*, based upon Otto Kernberg's (b. 1928) classification. I have my misgivings about such classifications, especially as they seem to be quite fluid and change often enough. The changes in such classifications are often for reasons other than clinical ones and have to do with market forces and fashionable ideas.

Still, I mention the diagnosis here as a cautionary note. We sometimes get blinded by such classifications and fail to see the intricacies involved. Often, we hide behind such classifications to explain away our own shortcomings in dealing with certain human behaviour that is perhaps beyond the scope of what psychotherapy can achieve. The fact that not all people can benefit from psychotherapy is not their fault but rather points out that psychotherapy is after all just one way of dealing with human suffering and does not always succeed. The following story is one of such a failure.

Having a fragmented sense of self, it is difficult to have a history which is not also fragmented. Amanda revealed parts of her biography to me begrudgingly, as this was often perceived by her as a sign of weakness and of losing control, of admitting to a willingness to fully participate in the sessions beyond just sitting there. My curiosity to know more was used by her as a reason to further withdraw, so I learnt to mute that part of me but to also leave a crack so that she knew I was there. My curiosity, even when not expressed through questions of any kind, but simply with a nod, a tilt of the head, a smile, were experienced by her as if they were direct assaults.

Amanda was a single 41-year-old Jewish woman when she began therapy. She was born in Birmingham, UK, and arrived with her parents to Israel when she was 2 years old. She had only ever left the parental home for very short periods and had been unemployed for most of her adulthood. She was an only child. Both her parents were in their late sixties when she first began therapy.

She grew up in a home of marital conflicts and deceptions. Her father conducted a long-term and stable extra-marital affair with a man whom most of the extended family had come across in various circumstances. Although this affair had never been formally acknowledged by the parents, it gradually became common knowledge, though silenced, and in a sense integrated into their family picture.

Amanda held a very affectionate view of her father as being a kind and warm man. She felt that he showed her more love than he did towards anyone else and felt safer when he was home, which was not often. Amanda's mother exercised a disciplinary style of parenting, watching Amanda's every move and always finding fault in her actions.

Amanda was a precocious child who suffered strong mood swings that often caused her trouble at school. She managed to perform above average in her schooling until she was 14 years old, which is when she tried to kill herself by drinking a large quantity of cleaning materials. She was found on the bathroom floor and was revived by her father. She was not taken to the hospital but stayed at home to recover. When her schoolteacher asked about her, it was reported that she had the flu.

When Amanda was 19 years old, she made her second suicide attempt after an intense fight with her mother. Her fear of her mother was so great that even after she woke up in hospital, having had her stomach pumped clean of the 40-odd tablets that could have killed her, she claimed that she had wanted to die because of unrequited love.

There were big gaps as to what had transpired with her in the years preceding her arrival at the out-patient psychiatric unit at the local hospital in Tel Aviv one Wednesday afternoon in March 1999. She came up to the counter, presented a referral letter from her GP and said that she wanted an experienced male therapist because she did not want to waste any time nor would she be able to trust a woman therapist. I had been working at that clinic for several years and was asked to see her for an initial assessment.

When I first met her, she immediately began interrogating me about my experience and expressed some concern as to whether I could be of any use to her as I looked too young. This took some time and when I commented upon the anxiety she might be feeling in the first session, she relaxed a little bit and spent some time looking at me and at the room with an intense and worried look on her face.

She then took out of her handbag a list she prepared with all the issues she wanted to go over in her therapy. She began reading from it: she felt dissatisfied with the kind of relationships she had with men; she was dissatisfied with jobs she had had in the past; she felt at a crossroads in her life; and she wanted to live away from the parental home. She read the list quickly and mechanically. She then stopped and expressed a worry that I would get depressed if I listened to her anymore. With some encouragement, she continued telling me about what had brought her to seek therapy at this time, including her suicide attempts and her sense of having failed at what she had hoped to achieve in her life. She kept interrupting herself and asked whether I thought I could help her and whether I was not bored with her.

Her speech was very fast, fragmented, and highly associative. She obviously had to control a lot of thoughts and feelings. Later, I came to understand that her recurrent queries regarding how I would be affected by her material was an indication of things to come. I thought she was still anxious and misinterpreted her remarks as showing some degree of self-awareness, therefore providing a good indication for starting therapy.

A few weeks later, Amanda entered the room enraged about how she was spoken to by the secretary of the clinic. When I responded in a reassuring way, like my tone in the first meeting, she turned her rage towards me and accused me of being unemphatic, cruel, too young, and in cahoots with the authorities. I was taken by surprise. I had thought that some trust had been established during the first sessions but realized that it was built on very shaky ground.

I began to consider that perhaps I was totally wrong in how I understood her. I spoke about that with my supervisor, and it was becoming clearer that we were not sharing the same *framework* as I had hoped. My psychoanalytical supervisor, who was far more experienced than me at that time, suggested that while my mental framework was verbal, she was employing a quite different framework, built upon a more idiosyncratic code of transformation of experience, a more peculiar personal mode of overcoming chaos and securing the indispensable backdrop or frame of mental existence. She thought that in this case it was not an imagined or fantasized antagonism but an actual power struggle over the way meaning is to be established and understood between Amanda and me. The task of establishing a common framework between us needed to be of the highest priority, more than the uncovering of the unconscious or the analysis of the self, the ego defences, or the transference and resistance.

It took me quite a long time to understand how poorly I was using my supervisor's valuable insights. Only years later, I thought that perhaps Amanda was right in the first place: perhaps I was too young and not experienced enough then.

The following session, she threw a fit for the first time in my presence. It seems to have come out of the blue. I was stupefied and for a long time remained silent. It was as if she was alone in the room. It was a blind narcissistic rage, directed towards a nonexistent or destroyed object. After a few minutes, when I tried to remain alive by speaking aloud, she seemed to wake up from a stupor, take notice of me, and was able for a very brief and lucid moment to acknowledge her desperation and frustration at getting so worked up and losing control.

She showed what I again mistook for an insight. After remaining quiet for a minute or so, she looked at me directly and confided with no apparent reason that she felt she used sex as a way of relieving tension in herself but was ultimately unsatisfied. I was surprised but tried to rise to what I thought was a meaningful moment by saying it must feel frustrating to want to connect with a man and feel that she could do this only through sex. Her response caught me off guard. She denied angrily and again seemed to get into a fit of verbal insults, saying that I was wrong, that I misunderstood her. She felt hurt and isolated. She then said that she thought that the therapy was not helping her at all and that she did not know whether she was going to come again.

In supervision and in my own therapy, I allowed myself to admit to feeling overwhelmed. I was indeed a young man, still unmarried, and Amanda's explicit sexual innuendos did feel provocative in a sense I found hard to contain. When my supervisor asked me point blank whether I felt sexually attracted to Amanda, I was not taken aback. Amanda was indeed attractive, and I noticed that when she first entered the room. That initial attraction faded quite quickly as I got to know her and her predicament. My supervisor wisely commented that Amanda might be reacting to my rejection of her as a woman and therefore was trying her best to win me back, as it were. She also advised me strongly against making an interpretation based upon such a suggestion as it would be seen as very intrusive by Amanda. All I could do, she thought, was to contain the situation and hope that a new form of *epistemic trust* would be formed with Amanda. What helped me at that time was realizing that I was not really dealing with a mature woman but rather with a young little girl who was trying to make contact but failing time after time. My supervisor thought Amanda was acting up like a 5-year-old girl would. She was attempting to seduce me into an abusive relationship, which was perhaps an echo of what really went on with her beloved and tantalizingly absent and intrusive father.

Erotic Transference

Over the next few months, it seemed that each session was a version of its predecessor. She would come into the room, sit down, tell me that she was tired or bored, and provide some anecdote about a date she had had during that week or some exchange with her parents. When I responded to whatever she had just said, attempting to be attuned to what I sensed was her mood, she dismissed my words as inadequate, cold, cruel, and irrelevant. And without fail, after a few minutes of such an attack, she would slump back into her chair and remain silent. With her eyes buried in the carpet, she would then suddenly announce that the session was over and leave the room, regardless of how much time remained.

A few weeks later, she began trying to cancel sessions by ringing the clinic and saying she could not bring herself to attend as she was not feeling well. She would engage the secretary in long conversations and somehow persuade herself to arrive after all. When I asked her about that, she became coy and evasive and insisted that she wanted to have a break from therapy in a manner which was both pleading and threatening. At other times, she spent most of the session lashing out at me for various inadequacies in the way the clinic was being run, the way the room was decorated, my manner of greeting, and more. These attacks were followed by apologetic telephone conversations with the secretaries, asking them to check whether I was angry with her. The problematic nature of these telephone conversations, which at first I thought constituted some attempt at reparation but offered various questionable excuses, became clear to me as they increased in frequency and seemed to constitute the bulk of the interaction over a period of several weeks when Amanda did not show up for her sessions.

Considering my supervisor's advice, I wondered whether a therapeutic alliance had been formed or perhaps was just a false one. I worried that my optimism that I was able to contain her was in fact doing the opposite. Was my *containment* of Amanda experienced by her at that stage as a trigger, as getting too close? Was what I thought of as containment experienced as an attack, an infringement of her boundaries, against which she had to fight?

I diligently but unsuccessfully tried to arrange the following sessions at Amanda's convenience. During the fifth month of therapy, after missing two sessions and ringing numerous times, she arrived at the scheduled meeting. She entered the room in a seemingly relaxed manner and began recounting in detail stories about her sexual activities, which involved having sex with men she knew, one of which was her ex-boyfriend, now married to someone else.

She took her time and lingered in her descriptions, provocative in her choice of words. She also paused frequently, giggled as if in embarrassment, and kept asking if it was okay that she told me such details. I hardly had any time to respond, indeed feeling quite at a loss as to where I should direct a response, to her teasing content or the anxiety I felt that lay beyond the stories. Seeing my hesitation, she became very alert and waited.

I felt I was entering a trap, told her so, and responded that her stories were indeed highly explicit and that I knew that there wasn't a straight answer to her question. I confessed that I felt she wanted to shock me, and she had succeeded, but nevertheless, I remembered her stress and pain from having such sexual encounters in the past. I dared to go a bit beyond my supervisor's advice.

My words were met by a flat denial and then anger at being misunderstood. Her denial was quick. I was indeed slightly embarrassed and not sure what path to follow. An awkward silence followed. I felt as if anything I might say was wrong and suggested to her, after inquiring what she was thinking about and facing a flat rebuff, that she did not want me to say anything as this interrupted her fantasy. She seemed to be submerged in private thoughts. She said that the silences were uncomfortable for her and began expressing concern that she was being listened to by someone outside the room and even checked by looking out into the corridor. Yet, she kept silent and would not respond to my comments, which tried to focus on the embarrassment she might be feeling. The session ended after a few minutes when she just got up and left without saying a word, well before the time was due.

High Noon

Without understanding exactly why, she reminded me of a film I loved, *High Noon*.

High Noon (1952) tells the story of Marshal Will Kane, played by Gary Cooper, possibly the ultimate masculine model of those times, a man who does not show emotions and never speaks but does the right thing, who stays in town to face a dangerous outlaw even though everyone abandons him. On the day he is supposed to retire and leave with his new wife, Kane learns that Frank Miller, a man he once arrested, is returning on the noon train for revenge. Kane knows that if he leaves, the outlaw will destroy the town. He tries to gather help, but one by one the townspeople refuse. Even his deputies and friends make excuses, leaving him to face the danger alone.

I admired that film and Kane's decision as it was based on what I believed to be an inner moral code. He feels he cannot run away without betraying both his role as marshal and his own sense of self. This makes him deeply isolated. He walks through empty streets, hearing only the sound of the ticking clock as noon approaches. His loneliness shows the cost of choosing principle over safety.

I thought that Kane's struggle was a battle between fear and duty, or between instinct and conscience. Freud described this tension as the conflict between the *id* and the *superego*. Kane's *ego* must find a path between these pressures. His decision to stay, even when abandoned, shows the strength of his superego; he cannot escape the law he carries inside himself.

When waiting for Amanda, I felt like Gary Cooper, mentally walking the deserted streets and wondering where I would find help for myself so that I could help her. I knew without doubt that her pain was real and huge. She rang the clinic several times during that week and demanded to speak with me. During the first couple of months of therapy, I used to reply to her calls empathetically, believing them to be signs of her neediness, and therefore responded from the position of wanting to provide holding. It was also the agency's policy. It took me a while to realize that what Amanda was trying to do, and to an extent accomplished, was to subtly change the terms of our dialogue so that it could be conducted over the telephone while she was ensconced in her bedroom. This became clear after a fortnight of missed sessions for which she offered various excuses, all the while trying to talk with me on the phone every day. When I made it clear that I was not going to respond to her telephone calls and that anything she wanted to say would have to be said within the session hour, she appeared for the next session and told me in great length, with a triumphant smile on her face, about all the sex calls she had been engaging in at that time. It was clear that she was feeling victorious in having fooled me.

During the next session, after starting by blaming the government for her poverty and inability to find a job, she suddenly calmed down and proceeded to take out a box from her bag, open it, and take out a large vibrator, pointing it in my direction and asking me to hold it. I was stunned. Eventually, I asked her what she expected me to do, and she replied that she wanted me to experience what she was entertaining herself with. She added, giggling, that she also wanted me to see her in her sexy underwear so that I could get "a true impression" of what she was really like. When I commented that the best thing we could do was discuss what she had hoped to achieve with such a proposal, she objected and claimed that I did not understand her. A few minutes later, she got up and left, placing the vibrator into her bag but leaving the box behind.

I felt a mixture of fear and anger as to what would follow. I remembered the advice I received of how important it was not to defend myself too strongly against the psychotic components of the transference. I was swamped, trying to survive but getting a sense that I was not doing so well.

As much as I tried to resist her attacks upon me, I felt that I was being reduced to a position of incompetence and helplessness. I tried to share with her how scary it must have felt for her to be under attack, and Amanda responded with derision and denial. In my supervision, I expressed my sense that I was doing really badly as a therapist and perhaps should terminate the therapy.

The next few sessions were taken up by Amanda flooding the therapeutic space with her erotic fantasies about me. This took the shape of disjointed talking interrupted by giggling and denials, interspersed with spells of anger directed at me.

My attempts to interpret what was going on met with either flat denial or juvenile glee, as if she had succeeded in achieving her purpose, i.e. to incorporate me into her sexual fantasies. This often gave way to paranoid fear. She would be convinced that someone was listening in on the sessions. With Gary Cooper seeking help from the community in mind, I began discussing with my supervisor the option of terminating the therapy and referring Amanda to a residential place where she would benefit from a wider array of therapeutic support.

An End?

Just as I was ready to give up and inform Amanda of that option, she arrived in a quiet and serene mood and launched into a continuous monologue, leaving little space for me to do anything but listen. She spoke almost in a state of trance, sharing with me details of her fears. She told me of her horror of thunder. On a stormy night, she would lie in bed and listen to the thunder. Someone had told her that one could calculate the distance to the thunder by counting the seconds between the sound of thunder and the flash of lightning. Thus, she would both comfort and frighten herself by imagining the thunder getting closer. If she could tolerate the pressure no longer, she would get up and go to her parents' bedroom and ask to be let in for comfort. It was easy to feel tender empathy towards her. She seemed like the little girl needing comfort I had imagined her to be, and my words seemed to have worked. She stayed for the length of the session and thanked me at the end as she was leaving.

Alas, in the session that followed she denied, negated, ridiculed, and blew to smithereens all that seemed to have been said by her and by me. She seemed to truly convince herself, and nearly me too, of the worthlessness of the previous session, thus protecting herself from any possibility of future contact, with the attendant horror of possible rejection. I realized that Amanda needed to exhaust me in a sense before she allowed herself to share her concerns without feeling threatened.

It was time for me to write a report to the health authority to request that her treatment be continued, as is customary in public mental health settings. I felt a great urge to write the application in such a way that it would not be approved. I was fully aware that my negative transference here was at play as I was seeking an escape from continuing therapy as it was becoming harder and harder to bear her identifying me with a malicious and abusive object. Denying her further therapy would be an enactment on my part and would fulfil her deeply seated fear of being annihilated by someone close to her. At the same time, I was also aware that if I applied to extend her therapy beyond what was usually allowed in the public sector, she would know this and it might play into her erotic transference fantasies about me, which in turn would further increase her attacks on the setting of the therapy.

With some misgivings in my heart and after lengthy discussions with my supervisor and colleagues, I decided to try the impossible and write the report asking for her to be referred to a particular residential home in the North of Israel, which was renowned for being a good place. I argued that continuing in weekly individual ambulatory therapy was not the right course of action. Perhaps what Amanda would benefit from was a voluntary residence in a special therapeutic community which would both remove her from the toxicity of her home and allow for a greater containment of her turmoil. There were other facilities that would have been suitable, but they all had very long waiting lists. I discussed this with my supervisor, and we agreed that a way must be found to convey that information to Amanda in a manner that would not feel threatening and rejecting. We decided to include that suggestion in the report as a viable alternative to individual therapy.

Amanda of course was aware of the report being written, and we scheduled a special session where I shared with her the details of the request, referring to both options. I was expecting a storm in response, but none occurred. She said that she had been offered such residential care in the past and did not want it. She said she wanted to continue individual weekly therapy with me. She left that special session calmly, but the storm did arrive during the next sessions.

The next couple of months were dominated by turmoil. Amanda brought a copy of the report and tore it up in front of me. She also wrote a complaint to the director of the clinic. In the room, she hurled very severe verbal abuse at me and on two occasions physically threw things at me. She would then leave the room in fury when my comments, or silence, were too much for her and harangued the secretarial team of the clinic with daily phone calls, becoming gradually but surely the most feared client in the clinic. On one occasion she attempted to expose herself in the room.

I was often left in the room to deal with the debris of her acting out and internal turmoil. I felt exhausted by the internal work I had found myself conducting to contain my transference. It was hard to gain insights into her mental constitution while being attacked. I was feeling increasingly frustrated at not being able to use any of my insights and felt very lonely during the sessions in my attempts to maintain an empathic position towards her. I also knew beyond doubt that my attempts to hold the situation were essential and was confirmed in that by my supervisor.

The health authorities partially approved our request for further treatment, which meant she would have to contribute towards payment for future sessions. This was not unusual as she had been in fully subsidized therapy for some time. The public health system was undergoing changes; budgets were being tightened and thus many treatments were being minimalized. The request for a placement in a special facility was approved in principle but remained pending because of lack of a suitable place at that particular time.

Her response in the form of an outburst of rage did not surprise me. She then became somewhat coy and for the first time confessed her worry that she would not be able to raise the necessary sum. When the day of reckoning was getting near, Amanda failed to appear for what would have been the last three sessions, ringing in and apologizing. She asked the secretary to thank me and said that I had helped her a lot and that when she got a proper job she would return.

I Am a Failure

My supervisor tried to reassure me that it would be unrealistic to expect her to behave in any other way. She also reminded me of her previous suicidal attempts and thought that what I had been doing with Amanda had steered her clearer off that dangerous path. Still, I was experiencing a sense of loss. I was deeply moved by her solitary and incessant attempts to make contact, however perverted. My supervisor thought that a seed of hope had been planted in our meetings. I was not so sure of myself. I even began suspecting my supervisor of being too kind in a condescending way. I had a dream where I heard her whisper to the director of the clinic that I was a hopeless therapist. When I told her about the dream, we agreed that it was a healthy sign of my unconscious process of working out my sense of professional failure. She also suggested that it was a good sign of my journey of becoming a good-enough therapist.

This continued to haunt me for months. I kept hearing my own critical voice saying that I had not been able to help her deal with her inner turmoil. In less self-reproaching moments, I reminded myself that her character and behaviour had demanded of me high levels of restraint, boundary watching, and patience. I knew I was dealing with a person whose ability to enter, engage in, and maintain *a working therapeutic alliance* was very limited, and my work was mostly confined to protecting the shell of the therapeutic setting.

It appeared that the very offer of such a setting posed a threat and a challenge to the perverse way she had led her life. I felt I had been skidding on thin ice to protect her from the abyss of her internal turmoil and terrors. The bulk of the sessions were dedicated to a struggle between two forces. One was determined to perversely avoid dealing with the pain, which was the manifest reason for the therapy, and the other attempted to construct a bypass that would possibly allow a passage over the abyss.

On more than one occasion I found myself wishing for the therapy to end. Beyond the obvious informative function of such transference, I was also desperately grappling with existential questions as to whether it was at all feasible for someone suffering like this to stay in any relationship where so much anger and hatred were being evoked.

From the material Amanda presented through her words but more significantly through her actions, I thought she was enacting and repeating early faults and holes in the maternal matrix. Often, it felt that immediately upon meeting me Amanda would "vomit" herself into the session by means of violent and venomous eruptions over which she had no control. It was as if the mere offer of contact threw her off balance, as would often happen to her in her life, whereby any man she had a slight attraction to would soon be "flooded" with her inappropriate sexual innuendoes, therefore contaminating her own intentions.

I believe that she showed what Winnicott would describe as a failure in *normal emotional development*. He wrote about how infants should be able to slowly and gradually develop separate expressions of aggressive and erotic components. The parent's, or the therapist's, role is to hold each separately for the client, who, in the transference, cannot survive an integration of the two. Such a failure to integrate results in the client's relationship with the therapist as being alternatingly aggressive and erotic.

Amanda's acting out in the *transference* can be understood as a kind of memory. What she was evoking and bringing to life through her tempestuous and tantrum-like behaviour was the failure of an early containment of her primary mental life. I was being cast repeatedly in the role of the abusive, tantalizing, seductive, and punitive parent. I felt desolate in my repetitive failure to support and repair the containing setting of the therapy which Amanda felt compelled to ferociously attack. On the rare occasions she allowed herself a respite – the sessions when she related her deeply felt and seemingly psychotic fears – Amanda seemed to use me as a paternal object, passive and weak, unable to penetrate the world of horror she was describing and feeling powerless to do anything but acquiesce in her pattern of only feeling safe with a distant, non-sexual, uninvolved male.

Amanda's treatment was ended by her, reflecting the pattern of all relationships she had been involved in. I could not help feeling partially responsible for that ending. Perhaps I had been too young and inexperienced. I was left wondering whether she was able to gain some insight from therapy or that it was just another link in a long chain of futile attempts at human interaction.

What she was able to do was let me in on her current incapacity to share without being destroyed. She was still organized mentally around the notion of ruthlessness, a far cry from having any capacity for concern. Only the passage of time will tell whether this therapeutic trial was a small step forward or just another representation of Bollas' grossly *traumatic dissonant attunements* continuously enacted throughout her adulthood with other people as her accomplices.

Reflecting back, I realize that weekly individual psychotherapy was indeed not enough. Amanda needed more than that. She deserved more than that. Once a week just wasn't enough when it came to trying to heal the catastrophic emotional damage she suffered. It was an important lesson for me regarding the capacity of any one therapist in dealing with such enormity of pain. There is an old proverb saying that it takes a whole village to raise a child. I believe that it is relevant to the attempt to help someone in Amanda's position. It would take a whole community to help her resurrect her damaged self. She herself was like Gary Cooper walking the deserted streets seeking support.

I left the out-patient clinic about a year later, so I had no idea as to whether Amanda did find a way into such a community. My role in her journey was a brief one, and I was left with a lot of questions marks regarding the outcome.

Beyond the unique characteristics of this case, such an ending is not unusual. There are many aborted therapies which leave therapists wondering what evolved in their clients' lives. This is one of the less favourable aspects of therapeutic work. For a time we are invited into someone's life and become involved. If all goes relatively well, we are able to complete a journey, or a significant part of it, so that the end of the therapy does not feel like a rapture. We are able to participate in a mourning process to enable a good-enough parting which is beneficial to both parties.

This was not the case with Amanda. Ending a therapy like that leaves both parties at risk of having unprocessed injuries. In the case of the therapist, this injury can and needs to be worked out in supervision. The client, on the other hand, is often left alone, having experienced another aborted attempt at making meaningful human contact.

Our professional, ethical boundaries do not allow us to follow up with these people and check in on how they are doing. We are left dithering between a hope that they did find another therapeutic capacity and the despair that they have reverted to the old pathological defences. There is no happy ending. There is not even a good-enough ending. In the process of developing as a psychoanalytic psychotherapist, there is no bypassing the mourning such moments bring.

Mourning such narcissistic injuries and learning from them is a vital part of the journey and needs to be acknowledged. Such acknowledgement will allow us to continue rather than suffer in silence and slowly lose hope in the pursuit of what we do. As I repeat throughout this book, one of the mottos that has supported me in my work is the idea that *despair is not an option*, or as the proverb in the Jewish Pirkei Avot tractate (the ethics of the Fathers) says: *you are not obliged to complete your mission, but you are not permitted to stop trying while being alive.*

Chapter 6

The Secret Wound of Exile

Literature and Film as Analytic Third in Psychoanalytic Therapy

This chapter continues my exploration of *transference*, which I see as central in the practice of psychotherapy. In many ways, I see the interpretation of transference and its vicissitudes as the pivotal axis upon which psychoanalytic psychotherapy revolves. It is certainly one of the distinguishing factors which differentiates it from other forms of therapy. Transference in my opinion occurs in all forms of therapy, as well as in life outside the consulting room, but it is only in psychoanalytic psychotherapy that it is given its proper weight.

Transference is the medium through which the therapist experiences the significant repetition of what the client unconsciously brings to therapy. It is not a simple linear repetition but an elaboration of past patterns which manifests both the way the client and the therapist *connect* and the way they are held *separate* by their uniqueness. The play between these two intertwined elements, *connection* and *separateness*, and their reappearance in the therapeutic relationship create the space wherein therapeutic change can take place. Such space will allow an evolving change in the client's capacity to deal with past stressful events so that they are no longer bound by pathological defence mechanisms. In other words, a positive outcome of therapy is when the client is freer to engage in their present relationships and in their creative and professional pursuits.

Exile: Connection and Separateness

Quite a few of the chapters of this book study the notion of *exile* in various forms, both inside the therapeutic room and in literature. I view exile, real and metaphoric, as one of the defining paradigms of our culture. I begin this study of exile with a short reference to Freud which I will delve into more extensively in Chapter Nine. Freud's exile from Vienna in 1938 was an individual event which also signified the exile of the psychoanalytical movement. He escaped the Nazi regime with ten members of his family. Freud could not save all his own family. His four sisters and their families were left behind and were murdered by the Nazis and their allies amongst 6 million Jews. Overall, the Nazis and their allies were responsible for the murder of 11 million people

DOI: 10.4324/9781003683162-6

through systematic genocide, war crimes, and mass persecution. Amongst the victims were many members of my own maternal family in Greece and France. I wrote extensively about that in my 2021 book, *Post-Memory, Psychoanalysis and Holocaust Ghosts: The Salonica Cohen Family and Trauma Across Generations.*

Freud reached England, where he died *in freedom* a year later. Freud's experience of exile reflects and resonates with the centrality of the exile experience in the 20th century. It was an exile both from his native land as well as a figurative exile from his psychoanalytic project. One of Freud's aims in his psychoanalytic project was to scientifically find salvation for man's tortured soul. He hoped that using the rational means of analysis would facilitate that. In a way, his exile and flight from the Nazis' evil forces of irrationality was bitter proof of the futility of his universal claims.

The correspondence between Ernest Jones (1879–1958) and Anna Freud (1895–1982) during the exile years in London highlights Freud's personal peril exile as the hallmark of our time, serving as both a reminder of the darkest times as well as a warning. A warning regarding the fragility of our sense of freedom, which can be shattered easily either by external or internal circumstances. Once that sense of freedom is lost, one faces a choice of giving in to despair or trying to regain it. Freud had to be exiled away from his beloved native land to maintain his freedom. Paradoxically, of course, he was no longer able to enjoy a true sense of freedom once his links to his native land were severed. Exile granted him physical freedom but at a cost. What I take from that last episode of his life is that one cannot give in to despair and must continue to strive to achieve what has been an authentic motive in one's life: the struggle for freedom and truth. It is a constant struggle that cannot by definition end. The actual struggle can be held as a flag and a sign by which the individual is guided. Giving up such a struggle is akin to giving in to one's defensive fears, which inhibits us from conducting a full, collaborative, and creative life with our fellow human beings. Viktor Frankl (1905–1997) and Bruno Bettelheim (1903–1990) are two examples for excelling in such a struggle.

Frankl and Bettelheim both survived the Holocaust, and their survival shaped the way they thought about life and creativity. Frankl, who was a psychiatrist, endured years in Nazi concentration camps. In those terrible conditions, he discovered that people who could find meaning in their suffering were more likely to survive. Out of this insight, he later developed *logotherapy*, a form of therapy that helps people search for meaning in their lives, even in pain and hardship. For Frankl, creativity became a way to affirm life, and writing, teaching, and helping others gave purpose after so much loss.

Bettelheim, a psychologist, also survived imprisonment in camps. His survival, like Frankl's, was tied to inner strength and the ability to imagine something beyond the horror. After the war, he turned towards studying children, especially those facing trauma or autism. He believed that stories, imagination, and symbols could help children make sense of their inner worlds.

For both men, survival was not just about staying alive. It was about transforming unbearable suffering into creative work that could heal others. Their experiences showed that even in the darkest times human beings can turn pain into new ways of understanding life.

Everyday Exile

It is common today to say that we are all in exile and that it is the basic condition of the modern person. While this is indeed a well-worn subject, it still deserves consideration. We are exiled from our mother's womb, from our childhood, from imagined happiness, from peace of mind. All of this describes our state of being in exile, even when we have not moved anywhere away from our homeland.

The term is evidently riddled with individual and collective connotations revolving around the moving, uprooting, resettlement, and deportation of individuals and groups of people. There are several alternatives that can be used to describe that momentous shift in one's link to one's place of origin and belonging, such as emigration, moving away, travelling, and, in Hebrew, *Aliya*, denoting specifically the act of Jews immigrating to the modern state of Israel. Presently in Israel, we are witnessing the massive relocation and possible future exile of thousands of Palestinians within the Gaza strip as the result of the ongoing war which broke out after the 7th October Hamas attack. Each term carries within it different connotations, sometimes telling a different story.

Narratives of exile, whether individual or collective, self-inflicted or enforced, may have at least one factor in common: the change in one's relation to one's place of birth, residence, or belonging. Such a change can be traumatic or liberating, or perhaps a mixture of both polarities. Being primarily a term used to describe one's cultural and social bearings vis-à-vis one's relation to one's homeland, exile can be easily misconceived as relating only to concrete, earthly circumstances and therefore not an obvious target for psychoanalytic investigation. Nevertheless, it is a potent term, central to one of psychoanalysis's most prevailing metaphors, *the oedipal complex*.

The theme of being exiled, and the symbolic and concrete consequences of that exile, resonates throughout that myth. Oedipus was exiled from his home and family and homeland so that he could be spared a tragic life and yet found his way back and indeed suffered the very dire consequences that were prophesized for him. One cannot escape one's fate.

Exile is one expression of the human capacity for mobility. Mobility is an important element in humanity's adaptive capabilities. Moving away from and returning to one's home is part of the human endeavour to explore the growing relationship between oneself and the environment, as well as one's sense of identity. This positive outlook on moving away as an expression of asserting the individual's sense of independent and discrete identity does not romanticize exile and acknowledges the hardships experienced by the exile: solitude, estrangement, different languages, the prospects of unemployment, and other challenges.

The exiled individual is always conflicted, carrying what Julia Kristeva (b. 1941) named as their *secret wound*. They idealize all new aspects and experiences in the society of their new home while simultaneously devaluing the people and places they have left behind, regarding them as persecutory. This inner conflict is often managed through disassociation, which helps to avoid the mourning, remorse, and depressive anxieties that would otherwise be triggered and intensified by the migration, especially if it was undertaken voluntarily.

Experiences of separation can also help people grow. They allow us to develop the ability to be alone in a creative way while still being able to form meaningful relationships with others. Our personality develops partly through this balance of being connected to others but also knowing how to stand apart from them.

However, when separation is forced, or when it happens before a person is ready, it can cause harm and even trauma. The impact depends on timing and intensity.

This raises a question about exile. If exile, whether chosen or forced, feels like a tearing apart rather than just a moving away, then it should be understood as traumatic. Exile in this sense breaks the flow of time and space in a person's life and leaves deep psychological wounds. In such cases, instead of leading to growth or creativity, exile is more likely to produce symptoms that show lasting injury.

The exiled individual will simultaneously find and rediscover themselves in their new habitat. In a sense, they recreate their old territory in the new one, synthesizing the old with the new, acting upon the force of *repetition compulsion*. Whether they are forced away from their native land or choose to leave it, they will find that they carry it within them like a seed. Once settled in a new land, it will grow and root itself in such a way that enables the diligent observer to examine its origins.

In the following pages, I shall place the theoretical issues I have discussed within the fictional case study of David.

Epistemic Trust

David arrived one afternoon for an appointment he had made over the telephone a few days earlier. When he rang to inquire whether he could make an appointment, he sounded cheerful. He asked whether I was the same person as the author of an article concerning writing and psychotherapy. I responded briefly and affirmatively, and he sounded pleased and reassured. After putting the phone down, I made a note to myself about his soft accent, which I could not quite place.

I wondered about his knowledge of my writing, but as it wasn't the first time a client has read something I had written, fiction or non-fiction, I felt quite at ease about it. From experience, I have learnt that once the initial interest in my writing subsides, it does not change the course of therapy in a very significant way. Once clients arrive at my clinic and see that the walls are lined with books, they accept my interest in writing as a natural extension of who I am and stay focused upon their own issues.

David was a very tall man with a beaming face. Immediately upon seeing him, taking visual note of his height, and hearing his soft Argentinian accent (which I recognized this time), I was reminded of Julio Cortázar. Cortázar was an Argentine writer whose work I loved and had read throughout my life. At first, I considered this to be a transference experience, whose meaning would become clearer later as the therapeutic relationship developed.

That very first time he entered the room, I noticed that his handshake was firm and warm and lingered ever so gently, as if he was waiting for my signal before releasing his grip. I note these very early impressions not just as a prelude to what followed but also as containing information regarding stages of *attunement* and *pre-verbal signals* echoing our unconscious-to-unconscious communication.

When David began to speak, after a minute of hesitation, during which he looked around my office, letting his gaze linger upon the rows of books lining one of the walls, his voice had a slightly different quality. It was no longer the soft caressing wave that I heard over the phone. An edge was present, and I could also tell from his minute restlessness that he was being more careful now that he was talking in my presence. It was as if the actual meeting with me introduced an element of stress, putting him on his guard, guiding him to measure his words more carefully, reining in his initial enthusiasm and what seemed initially to be his good spirits.

I could feel that during those very first moments of the meetings with David I was invited to experience both his unique *idiom* and his *defences.* I wondered how that would influence the establishment of *epistemic trust* between us.

David spoke of a deep sense of dissatisfaction in his life. He has been working in a clerical job that he hated. He was married to a woman whom he felt no longer loved him. They had two sons and a daughter, whom he adored but who were closer to his wife. He said he thought he was experiencing *"an ordinary late mid-life crisis."* That last remark was uttered with self-derision.

He continued: *"Who doesn't complain about his wife, his job, life in general, at my age? It's pathetic. Thankfully, I no longer live in Argentina, so I don't have to fear complaining about the government"*.

Apart from relating his daily preoccupations concerning the mundane travails of his life, he told me of his family's hasty immigration to Israel during the late 1970s, when they had to flee their home in Rosario in fear for their lives, as did most of the Jewish community in the country.

He viewed the move to Israel as a blessing and as an act which saved his life. When he related his aggravation concerning his wife's lack of understanding and her judgemental attitude towards him, he sounded bitter, harsh, and forlorn. It was as if he had given up hope. He also sounded forlorn when we discussed his situation at work or his relationships with his children. I was experiencing him as addressing a paternal figure in me, seeking guidance and console in a world he felt had betrayed him.

When he reminisced about his childhood in Rosario, his manner would change quite dramatically. His eyes would assume a dreamy gaze as if he was watching some event occurring far away, or deep inside him. The change also altered his voice. His voice would become deeper, and his accent would be more pronounced. While talking about his childhood, his friends, and family events, he seemed happy.

He almost seemed like a different version of himself, *a Doppelgänger*.

His stories of his childhood and youth grew more detailed, and he confided in me accounts of very moving events. I was struck by the accuracy and the abundance of details of his tales. He had an extraordinary sense of detail and was able to recapture whole scenes and bring them back to life in the sessions. I was slowly following his mental journey back to his homeland, reconstructing with him the lost scenes of childhood.

While there was no actual change in David's current life situation and his marital and occupational difficulties remained objectively the same, the manner of reporting about them indicated that his subjective experience had altered. I felt that we had established *epistemic trust*. He sensed my willingness to learn from him and that gave him further permission to confide more in me.

Both in terms of volume and in terms of intensity, he seemed less perturbed and burdened by the demands that his daily chores placed upon him. David commented upon this himself. After a while, he said that he felt he no longer needed therapy as he was feeling much better. He felt he had come to terms with his situation, and though nothing had changed, he no longer suffered.

We discussed the prospect of ending the therapy, but David continued to express his need to continue our weekly sessions. There was no faltering in his showing up for his sessions, and he kept his payments regularly and on time.

After a few weeks, he spent less time talking about the issues that troubled him at first and was mainly concentrating on what seemed to be a focused attempt to relive his past in Argentina. His memories grew more vivid and alive. He questioned his relatives concerning details he was not sure about. He re-established contact with old childhood friends and even dedicated considerable effort to tracking down some lost friends. He told me of parties he organized in his house, to which he invited the "Argentine Mob" as he called his friends and associates from Rosario.

He often talked about what kind of person he would have become had he stayed in Argentina. He related to that other version of his life as if it was as real.

By sheer coincidence, I happened to see a movie during that time that made me think of him. Movies have always been a great source of inspiration as a form of art that captures many ideas concerning human development that are dealt with in therapy. In fact, my preoccupation with films began many years before I began working as a therapist, during the same years that I began to write and listen to music. Therefore, I would pay close attention to themes that emerged from the movies I saw.

The film in question was *The One I Love.*

The One I Love: Self-Exposure

Charlie McDowell's film *The One I Love* (2014) begins as a quiet story about a troubled marriage. Ethan (Mark Duplass) and Sophie (Elisabeth Moss) are a couple whose relationship is unravelling. On the advice of their therapist, they retreat to a secluded country house to reconnect. What seems at first like a peaceful getaway quickly turns strange when they discover a guesthouse on the property. Inside, each encounters a seemingly perfect version of the other. These doubles appear more loving, more attentive, more ideal. As the weekend unfolds, desire and suspicion intensify, leading to a final confrontation in which Ethan and Sophie must decide whether to remain with one another or abandon their flawed relationship for the seduction of perfection. The ending, deliberately ambiguous, leaves Ethan apparently reunited with Sophie, though hints suggest he may have left with her double instead.

This ambiguity is not simply a narrative trick. It captures something Freud himself identified. We all have different versions of ourselves and of our relationships – a *Doppelgänger* – embedded deep in our unconscious, versions that leave traces behind.

The strange doubles that Ethan and Sophie encounter represent the projections of their desires. In the film, this fantasy becomes literal: Ethan finds a version of Sophie who is softer and more admiring, while Sophie meets a version of Ethan who is more attentive and confident. These doubles appear perfect because they mirror the unspoken wishes each partner harbours. But as Freud observed, fantasies built on projection are destined to collapse. The more we idealize the other, the more unbearable their real imperfections become.

This collapse is experienced in the film as something uncanny. The doubles look and sound exactly like Ethan and Sophie, yet they are not quite right. Their flawlessness itself feels alien, even threatening. The family home, which should be a place of safety, becomes frightening and uncertain. By the end of the film, *the uncanny* has shifted into everyday life: Ethan believes he has escaped with his wife, but subtle signs suggest that she may not be the "real" Sophie. The safe space of home is permanently altered, just as Freud suggested that the uncanny makes the ordinary feel charged with danger.

A further idea at play in the film which I found relevant is *repetition compulsion*. The doubles in *The One I Love* seem to offer Ethan and Sophie a chance to break free from their cycle of disappointment and conflict. If only they could stay with the *better* versions, everything might be easier. But this is an illusion. By the end, Ethan is left uncertain whether he has escaped the cycle or has merely stepped into a new version of it. The film suggests that there is no real escape from repetition through fantasy; change can only come from facing the difficulties of the real relationship, as we do in psychotherapy.

This is why the ending of the film is so powerful for me. It denies the viewer the comfort of knowing whether Ethan has returned with Sophie or her double. Instead, we are left in the same position as Ethan: caught between trust and doubt, between reality and fantasy. The film's message is not that true love is impossible but that it is always shadowed by uncertainty. As in therapy, we can never fully know the other person. We love not just who they are but also who we imagine them to be. To continue in love is to live with this tension.

In the end, *The One I Love* dramatizes a truth that psychoanalysis has long recognized: intimacy is never free of illusion. We are drawn to others not only for who they are but for what they represent to us, for the unconscious wishes and fears they carry on our behalf. The doubles make visible what usually remains hidden, the way we long for our partner to be someone else, and the way this longing distorts our view of them. The final scene, with its unanswered question, forces us to confront the unsettling possibility that the person we return home to is never exactly the one we think we love. In my mind, David's fantasy of his lost childhood was exactly that.

Even though that film resonated with David's journey in more than one way, I decided to keep my thoughts about it to myself. Somehow, I never found the right moment to share these thoughts with him. I knew that these thoughts enriched and deepened my attention towards his story but felt that there was no benefit to gain from sharing the actual details. It would have been, I thought, overburdening David with my preoccupation and would have amounted to *self-exposure*.

For me, there is a continuum of self-exposure that stretches from facts, such as mentioning having children, sharing cultural interests, to revealing something more personal and emotional, like saying I also felt anxious in a similar situation.

I believe that self-exposure is risky. If the therapist shares too much, it may overwhelm the client or shift attention away from their needs. The danger of *self-exposure* in therapy has been on my mind during these years. Many of my colleagues and indeed the bon ton of the community were leaning in that direction. Stemming from the sensible idea that transference thoughts belong to the therapeutic dyad, many therapists find it necessary to share thoughts while applying enough censorship as to their relevance to the client and the therapeutic process.

My strongest objection to sharing such thoughts is based on the idea that one can never know in which developmental position the client will be when we share that thought. We might be thinking that we are exchanging ideas on an adult level, but our client may well shift at that very point to a regressed position, therefore experiencing our innocent sharing as intrusive. For that reason, I generally choose not to share such content.

Furthermore, I have found that keeping such content to myself as part of my *reverie* has proven to be very fruitful. I can contemplate wanting to share something and that thought has changed my position in the *transference* paradigm. I have found that my private, unshared, associations have helped me to understand better what the client is talking about. There is no need to disrupt their flow but rather be aware of the fine adjustments in your transference position to become even more receptive and attuned.

This is a fine balance I have learnt to hold: at times keeping my free and private associations to myself and at other times, more rarely, sharing them after very careful deliberation. For instance, I never shared with Amanda, from Chapter Five, my association concerning Gary Cooper and *High Noon* as I felt certain that such an association would be like inviting her into an intimacy which would be quite harmful.

I believe that one of the factors that indicates when it is right to share the therapist's association is determined by the level of *epistemic trust*. If *epistemic trust* is well established, it also implies that the *therapeutic alliance* is sound and can contain such a sharing, done of course in a timely and compassionate manner. If epistemic trust is still developing, it is wiser to avoid such sharing lest it create a less desired outcome.

When the client says something that resonates with the therapist's own association, it can signify that it is beneficial to share that thought, as was the case with David and Cortázar, where I felt more at liberty to allow my thoughts to enter the conversation.

The Breakdown and the Dream

Just as I thought we were moving safely towards closure, a turning point occurred after a holiday break I took, followed by absence due to David being sick. As we were meeting once a week, it meant we did not meet for a month. That was the longest break we had.

When we met again, he appeared perturbed. He reported that his depression had returned. The atmosphere was heavy, and I wondered whether his recovery of previous months was false, *a flight to health*. I found myself wondering that if the break of four weeks caused such heavy regression, then previous progress was not authentic, a mere wishful thinking on my part.

When I asked him if he was disappointed, he stated that *"on the contrary, his meetings with me were like an oasis, a safe place where he felt at home like he hasn't for years"*. As the minutes passed, I could see that he was feeling better again, and I commented upon it, feeling somewhat relieved but also dubious as to the durability of that positive outcome of the session. We shook hands again upon his initiative at the end of the session, something that had not happened since the very beginning of the therapy.

In the following session, he related a dream. This was not unusual for him, but both the timing and the content of the dream were unique. He started telling the dream almost as soon as he walked through the door, as if he had to share it with me but also as if he was afraid that he would lose it. I felt that I had to be very attentive and hold the dream like a treasure.

> *I arrived at your room after a very long journey which involved travelling overseas. It took me several days, and I had to change flights as well as board several trains in between. [With] each such boarding, taking off, and landing, I got lost and needed to ask for assistance along the way.*

He used repeatedly the verb *return* in the dream in many different contexts. He concluded the dream by saying that when he arrived I wasn't there.

He then stayed quiet for a very long time. As I was waiting, I was reminded of a short story by Cortázar, *The Southern Thruway*, which described an incident where a traffic jam goes on for days. During that long stay, the passengers begin to experience hallucinations and imagine that the scenery is shifting around them while they remain stranded on the road.

When David spoke again, returning as it were to the room, he seemed in possession of a deep insight. He interpreted the dream himself. He began describing my clinic as the *home* he was once exiled from as a young boy. My absence felt just like that. He feared he was being exiled again, having again to abandon his past and self.

I began to appreciate that the familiar feeling he was experiencing while telling me his childhood memories evoked in him the sense of belonging that was severed by his family's escape to Israel. While the therapy went on, he was able to feel at home again. His sense of well-being facilitated the subjective improvement in his current life and even brought about the creative upsurge in his social life. The threat of the end of the therapy during my absence was experienced as a repetition of the exile.

David brought an extract from *The Diary of Andrés Fava* to my attention the following session. In his posthumously published book *The Diary of Andrés Fava* (2005), Cortázar describes in the form of a diary the thoughts of a young man, presumably Cortázar himself, contemplating the event of *exile.* He describes the imperceptible removal of all that was familiar, like a house that loses its furniture piece by piece – its curtains, its paintings – while the life of its inhabitants continues with no possible variation.

During the following sessions, David realized that the source of his recent unhappiness was the understanding that what had helped him in therapy could be lost as his home was once lost. He became aware that the source of his unhappiness which brought him to therapy was not the daily difficulties but rather the tearing apart at his source of well-being that being exiled was causing him.

The facilitating environment that the therapy offered him recreated within him the well-being that he had associated with his childhood and with the good-enough parenting he had experienced. It was as if the process of telling stories about his childhood helped to regenerate, recuperate, and create a good-enough sense of belonging.

Finding in Cortázar's words both solace and inspiration, both an audience and an oracle, David talked about the power of words to transform his life. Without referring to it, he was describing Cortázar's words as *speech acts*, as words loaded with significance far beyond their symbolic meaning. He was thinking of certain sentences that he remembered as transformative. John Austin (1911–1960) defines *a speech act* as an utterance that has a performative function in language and communication. For example, the proclamation *I do* uttered as part of the wedding ceremony is a speech act. These are not just words but words which have performative and even legal repercussions.

Using his own words and the words of his beloved Cortázar gave a concrete form to his *mourning* process. It was almost as if he was composing a litany for the loss of his childhood and homeland. Once that was recognized, he was able to begin parting from it.

David realized that the improvement in his feelings was a result of his being able to both recreate his initial belonging to Argentina, as well as come to terms with the harsh emotions associated with the exile from it. Once he understood that, he was able to deal with the impending ending of the therapeutic relationship. The process of mourning that was thus begun allowed him to transform his melancholy into mourning. He began mourning his repressed loss.

The process of mourning which characterized the end of David's therapy took many paths. Once he realized how deeply anxious he was vis-à-vis the prospect of losing the safe place he had in my presence, he was able to consciously deal with the loss of that safe place, his homeland, he had prior to his exile from Argentina.

He became aware of the anger he stifled towards his parents, whom he secretly blamed for not being strong enough to overcome the persecution they experienced during the regime of terror in Argentina. He recalled several moments when his father seemed to be on the verge of a collapse, hiding it from him in a jovial and masculine manner.

A memory surfaced from when he was only 11; returning home from school, he found his mother in a state of anxiety. She disappeared into her bedroom, emerging only once his father returned from work. It was a matter of weeks from that moment until they left Argentina.

David was amazed to discover that even though he was fully aware and remembered many details from that period, including many details about the political situation in Argentina and the circumstances that made them leave, it was only during therapy that he began to feel the emotions associated with those incidents.

It was during that time that he began to read Cortázar again. The reading of Cortázar's work for the second time, the first time having been in Argentina, was *a homecoming* for him. During the intervening years, the memory of Cortázar's texts sunk into the same oblivion that his emotions sunk into. Re-reading Cortázar was like re-reading his emotions.

Cortázar was born in Brussels during one of his Argentinian father's diplomatic missions. Julio's father left the family and never returned when little Julio was 6 years old. Cortázar and his mother returned to the Banfield neighbourhood of Buenos Aires soon after. Here he spent his childhood and youth until he left at the age of 37 for Paris, where he lived until his death in 1984. During the many decades he lived in Paris, Cortázar worked as a translator for UNESCO, a job that gave him the time he needed to write and the opportunity to travel to various places around the world as part of his work.

The circumstances of Cortázar's exile from Argentina were, of course, different in many historical respects from David's, yet he too felt betrayed by his homeland due to its political changes and therefore chose to leave. Unlike David, however, he was also able to return to it, at least symbolically. In his posthumously published novel *Final Exam*, written in 1950, about a year before he left Argentina, one of the characters says that you can only appreciate your culture after being removed from it.

As David's therapy neared its end, I returned to that book whose protagonist, an Argentine student, struggles with the culture he lives in. He feels trapped by it, realizing that even distance cannot free him, that culture lives inside the body and cannot be escaped. Yet he hopes that leaving will let him see it from afar, with more understanding.

David came to a similar realization. Exile was not just about loss or longing. In Israel, he discovered parts of himself hidden in Argentina: his Jewish roots and the pull of the promised land. Life in Rosario had obscured this, but once he was forced to leave, ambivalence surfaced, belonging to both places yet betraying each at the same time.

Therapy helped him see that distance can also bring closeness. Exile created a new inner space where he could carry both versions of himself, like Cortázar's student in Paris or my own youthful poem. For refugees, exiles, and immigrants, this liminal space allows them to hold onto both their old and new worlds at once.

Exile, then, is not about erasing one's culture but reshaping your relationship with it. In doing so, one can regain perspective, hope, and agency, and recognize that life itself has always been a form of unconscious exile.

The Analytic Third and the Secret Wound

It was then that I was finally able to put into perspective my initial thoughts when I first met David. The fact that I was flooded with thoughts concerning Cortázar and later of the film *The One I Love* was not just an ordinary instance of transference. I suggest that Cortázar's work, and the film, served as an expression of *the analytic third* between David and me, thus allowing the unconscious communication that served as the basis for the therapeutic process. One came into the open while the other remained a private object which nourished me without being communicated to David.

As Thomas Ogden (b. 1946) wrote, *the analytic third* can be viewed as resulting from the reverie that the therapist allows himself. *The analytic third* is an expression of *the reverie* concerning the ordinary, everyday details of one's own life that are often of great narcissistic importance to both the therapist and the client. It was my reverie upon Cortázar in the context of David's preoccupation, in conjunction with David's original interest in his work, which allowed for this instance of the analytic third to be formed.

Bion's concept of reverie refers to the mother's (or therapist's) receptive, empathic state of mind that allows them to contain and process the infant's raw emotional experiences, or beta elements. Through reverie, these unprocessed sensations are transformed into meaningful, thinkable experiences, *alpha function*, enabling the infant to develop a sense of reality and emotional regulation. In therapy, reverie becomes the therapist's open, intuitive listening mode, allowing unconscious communication from the client to be received, metabolized, and interpreted. Reverie is thus a basic element in the development of the capacity to think and symbolize, both in infancy and in therapy.

Cortázar and his work, which have existed as an object for me from an early age, were used in an unconscious way by David. It was Cortázar and my own meditations on exile that served as the platform for the unconscious-to-unconscious reverie between us, enabling both David to feel at home and for me to be used by him as an imaginary home.

On the other hand, my experience and thoughts of the film were also an analytic third, but one which I chose to keep private. As we recognize that the client might have parts of themselves hidden from us not as *resistance* but as a natural process to do with the *separation-individuation* paradigm, so we as therapists need to be able to hold parts of ourselves to ourselves so as not to overburden the client with what is not relevant to their growth. Working with the *transference* paradigm still means that everything that is taking place within therapy belongs to transference, but not all must be shared.

The sense of being-at-home, which received no explanation during most of his therapy, became threatened during my absence and revealed how precarious being-at-home really is. Having accepted that sensation without subjecting it to *transference interpretation*, I was able unconsciously to serve as *a facilitating environment* for David's engagement with his exiled state to emerge.

David's evocation of my interest in Cortázar's writings at the very beginning remained unanalysed, unspoken about, and not understood. Bollas's *unthought known*, throughout the course of therapy, placed me in a position where he was able to use me as a container and gradually bring to the fore aspects of himself which remained deeply buried. The crisis of my absence, which re-evoked for David the crisis of his exile and the repression of his associated emotions, allowed him to begin a process of *mourning*, thus revealing to himself and to the world creative powers embodied through his interest in the texts of Cortázar, which had served him as *transitional phenomenon* during his adolescence.

Could it have been any other film or piece of text that made that specific connection between David and myself? Or was there something specific in Cortázar's text and the film which served as the platform through which David was able to use me as an object and articulate that aspect of his personal *idiom*? This question cannot but remain unanswerable. It is not a matter of truth but rather of truth seeking and interpretation.

In terms of unconscious-to-unconscious communication, it was Cortázar's text that served to bring about that aspect of David's particular idiom into play. At the same time, without my own particular interest in Cortázar's writing, as well as my private impression of the film, I would perhaps not have allowed myself the sense of playfulness and ease-of-mind to generate in me.

Unconscious-to-unconscious communication is a dialogue, a unique exchange depending on both participants.

The exiled person carries their existential state buried deep underneath layers of functionality. Preoccupied by daily experience, they strive towards distancing themselves from that *secret wound*. Mostly, this is successful, and exiles are able to adjust. But when they don't, and when, according to Kristeva, adjustment is not necessarily such a desired developmental goal, the secret wound shows itself in the subject interactions with the world and through a certain disability they carry. Often, they express their secret wound through particular metaphoric uses of cultural objects, forming attachments which seem to be peculiar without the knowledge of their purpose.

I think that David's usage of Cortázar's work was an example of such an attachment. The figure of Cortázar was well-known in Argentina during David's adolescence and since. Having left his homeland and settled in Paris because of being persecuted by the authorities, Cortázar can be seen as an exile who was able to address his secret wound openly. Furthermore, his preoccupation with it became one of the major subject matters of his work. He expressed that not only through overt writings about political issues, though he did that too by writing about Cuba and the Sandinista revolution in Nicaragua and through his work in various UN committees. More relevant to this discussion is the fictional world he created through his short stories, novels, and poems, where he established a *fictional homeland* often populated with imaginary figures.

David used Cortázar in such a way as to articulate a part of his *idiom* through his relation to me in the room. My own thoughts concerning Cortázar upon first seeing David were evidence of the unconscious communication which took place between us. His almost immediate sense of *being-at-home* in my presence was testimony to the rapport we shared, which was threatened and severed when a break in the continuity of the therapy repeated and gave expression to his secret wound of having been exiled. Experiencing that crisis not just as a crisis occurring in the transference but an articulation of an instance of his idiom facilitated for David an opportunity to come to terms with and then mourn the event of being exiled with his family from Argentina.

I conclude this chapter with a poem I wrote 40 years ago. This will perhaps further illustrate the centrality of the idea of exile in contemporary culture.

Thoughts on Being a Voluntary Exile

Not being able to have steaming Falafel
made by the sweaty and hairy hands of the Polish Holocaust survivor,
Class of 1932, with the numbers on his arm,
each bite spiced with the buses' fumes as they emerge, howling,
from the central bus station in Tel Aviv,
delivering ecstatic children to all corners of the Promised Land.

I was 5 years old when Jerusalem was occupied and liberated again.
The city that had championed many and washed in the blood of even more
once again is claiming a bitter price for her liberation
by one army from the occupation of another.
As a 5-year-old, it didn't make a great deal of sense.

Days of turbulence that linger into months of dislocation.
Like the buried bud during the long, cold winter,
I too know that the time of thawing will come,
that the natural rhythm of life will not pass me by.
But a darkness of suspicion never lifts.
Dreading that out of the slumbers of Now
only rot and decay will evolve,
mocking the long months spent in long patience.

Here, the cities of the West sprawl out into green.
There, cities merely sprawl, abruptly reaching an invisible line
that I am forbidden to cross by conscience and fear.
Over there, the "countryside", is where the Palestinians grow our tomatoes.
Every time an Israeli bites into the juicy fleshy vegetable
he must think of the hand that buried the seed in the soil,
the same hand that would be holding a stone on the following day.
The same hand that could be lying dead, rubber bullet and all.

"Biting the hand that feeds" acquires a new meaning in the Moledet (Moledet is the Hebrew word for The Country of Birth).

It means, the Country of Birth, or more loosely, The Motherland.
But I was born here, in the West, in the not-so-green Stoke Newington.
So where is my Moledet?
Perhaps in Lom by the Blue Danube, where my dad spent his first 16 years?
Or in the spacious house in Salonica, where my baby Mum gazed onto the humid street?
Or is it in the dusty army camp on an arid hill somewhere near Jerusalem,
where I spent the bitterest Yom Kippur truly atoning the sins that made me a soldier?

The security guard at the Orthodox Synagogue in Nottingham didn't believe my Jewish authenticity, one grey Yom Kippur
as I stood outside, wrapped up, seeking warmth amongst my ancient "brethren".
I didn't have a ticket…
The recital of Shema Israel convinced them that I had no intention of blowing the place up
so I didn't get arrested by the bemused policeman,
who was looking forward to a bit of action on that dull day.
But I did not gain admission.
I spent the rest of the day trying to explain to a Gentile lover
why I still felt a part of the Jewish people.

And still, I know it is true:
There is a dream I share with some multitudes here and everywhere.
A dream, a memory, a hope, that it hasn't all been in vain,
the screams of the victims, the songs of the pioneers,
the whispered prayer of the believers, the outspoken anguish of the intellectuals,
that one day the Moledet for some shall not be an exile for others.

Chapter 7

When Fathers Fall Silent

Music as a Transitional Object in the Adolescent Response to Paternal Trauma

In this chapter, I shall explore *adolescence* as an expression of a boy's developing *ambivalence* towards his father, who is emotionally absent due to his own pain. I will also demonstrate the use of art as a medium, specifically Pink Floyd's *Wish You Were Here* and The Who's 1967 rock opera *Tommy.*

Therapy is a verbal method through which meaning is gained, often mutual, in the dialogue between therapist and client. Over the years of my practice, I have often found myself turning towards additional artistic forms when struggling to give meaning to what I was going through.

When I began doing that, I felt I was somewhat deviating from what had been transcribed throughout my training as the single means of communication in psychoanalytic psychotherapy. Gradually over the years, I allowed more of my artistic pursuits to enter the therapy room, where they have served as inspiration without in any way disrupting what I still believe to be the fundamentals of psychoanalytic psychotherapy, as discussed in the first chapters of this book.

Music and Adolescence

In his 1914 *Some Reflections on Schoolboy Psychology* essay, Freud refers to the boy's disappointment and ambivalence once he realizes his father is not the omnipotent figure he once believed him to be. Such a disappointment is a conscious event. It has, of course, a positive developmental aspect, as it leads, amongst other things, to the development of the boy's ability to further separate from his original objects of identification and seek his place in the world.

Of all the images of a childhood – which, as a rule, can no longer be remembered – none is more important for a youth or a man than that of his father, according to Freud. We know that the loss of his own father and the ensuing depression he developed was one of Freud's main motivations in analysing his own dreams, leading to his seminal work on dreams.

Young children typically view their parents as highly capable and admirable figures who seem to know everything and can handle any problem. This idealization is a normal part of early development, where parents naturally appear larger-than-life to small children, who depend on them completely.

DOI: 10.4324/9781003683162-7

However, children also begin to recognize that parents set boundaries and enforce rules that sometimes conflict with what the child wants to do. This creates mixed feelings; the child continues to love and respect their parent while also feeling frustrated by the limits they impose. These conflicting emotions, admiration alongside occasional resentment, are common and usually persist in some form throughout life.

During early childhood, a child's perspective begins to broaden significantly. As they interact more with peers, teachers, and other adults, they start to see their parents more realistically. They may notice that other adults have different strengths, or that their parents don't know everything after all. This recognition can be disappointing, especially if the child has maintained very high expectations.

Another significant realization during this period is that the child realizes they are not the sole focus of their parents' attention and affection. They begin to understand that their parents have relationships with each other and with other people – spouses, friends, colleagues, and potentially other children – that are as important and meaningful. The child discovers they must share their parents' love and attention rather than being their exclusive recipient. This awareness can trigger feelings of jealousy or insecurity, but it also represents an important step towards understanding that relationships involve multiple people with their own needs and connections.

This shift from *idealization* to a more balanced view represents normal psychological development. The child begins to see their parents as real people with both strengths and limitations, rather than as all-knowing authority figures. While this process can involve some disappointment, it's also healthy; it allows the child to develop their own identity and judgement rather than remaining dependent on idealized parent figures.

The way children navigate this transition, learning to maintain love and respect for their parents while also developing independence, often influences their approach to authority figures and relationships throughout their lives. Some children manage this shift smoothly while others may struggle more with the disillusionment or have difficulty finding the right balance between connection and autonomy.

These processes are common to boys and girls in relation to either parent. It does not make any sense any more to think of the exclusivity of the parent–child relationship in terms of gender identification only. *Oedipal disillusionment* can occur to a girl or a boy in relation to both or either of their parents. Realizing that the person whom they thought loved them the most also loves somebody else as much, and perhaps more, is something both boys and girls have to deal with in relation to either parent.

In this chapter, I focus on what happens to one particular boy in relation to his father as he enters adolescence, but I believe insights regarding girls and their relation to their parents can also be drawn.

In the following pages, I shall illustrate how two great rock albums of the 1970s became objects of culture in therapy. The following short synopses of these two very different works by British rock groups that share some very poignant themes will introduce the clinical description and discussion.

Tommy: A Rock Opera by The Who

The Who's rock opera *Tommy* (1969) presents a compelling narrative centred on paternal absence and its psychological consequences. The story follows Tommy Walker, a boy who becomes "deaf, dumb, and blind" after witnessing his father's apparent death and subsequent return, which results in the killing of his mother's lover.

The absent father motif operates on multiple levels throughout the work. Initially, Tommy's father is presumed dead in World War I, creating a literal absence that forces his mother into a new relationship. When the father unexpectedly returns, his physical presence paradoxically intensifies his emotional absence, and he becomes a source of trauma rather than stability. This return triggers the violent confrontation that catalyses Tommy's psychosomatic conditions, suggesting that the father's reappearance is more damaging than his absence.

The narrative structure reinforces themes of paternal inadequacy through Tommy's subsequent experiences. His parents, unable to cope with his condition, subject him to various failed treatments and eventually abandon him to exploitation. The father's inability to connect with or protect his son reflects broader anxieties about masculine authority and family stability in post-war Britain.

Tommy's eventual emergence as a "pinball wizard" and spiritual leader can be interpreted as compensation for the paternal void. His extraordinary abilities and later messianic role suggest an attempt to transcend the failures of the father figure. However, his ultimate rejection by followers mirrors his own abandonment, creating a cyclical pattern of paternal absence and inadequacy.

The rock opera's treatment of the absent father reflects broader cultural concerns about changing family structures and masculine identity in the 1960s. Pete Townshend's composition uses this central absence to explore themes of trauma, healing, and the search for authentic connection in a fragmented modern world. The work ultimately questions whether paternal absence creates opportunity for self-determination or perpetuates cycles of dysfunction and alienation.

Pink Floyd's *Wish You Were Here*

Pink Floyd's 1975 album *Wish You Were Here* explores the psychological fragmentation that results from external pressures and internal conflicts, serving as both a meditation on mental breakdown and a commentary on the music industry's dehumanizing effects. The work emerged during a period when the band witnessed their former member Syd Barrett's decline, making it a deeply personal examination of stress-induced psychological collapse.

The album's central narrative traces the gradual erosion of individual identity under systemic pressures. The work suggests that creative individuals are particularly vulnerable to mental deterioration when subjected to familial exploitation and societal expectations that conflict with artistic integrity.

The concept of "burning out" versus "fading away" becomes a crucial metaphor for different modes of psychological decline. The album presents stress not as a singular traumatic event but as a sustained pressure that gradually erodes cognitive and emotional stability. This process manifests through alienation from one's creative work, loss of genuine human connection, and the substitution of authentic experience with artificial constructs.

The work's sonic architecture reinforces these themes through extended instrumental passages that mirror psychological states. Repetitive structures and ambient soundscapes create a sense of mental circling and trapped consciousness, while sudden dynamic shifts represent moments of clarity or breakdown. The interplay between organic and synthesized sounds reflects the tension between authentic human experience and artificial social constructions.

Pink Floyd uses the absent friend as a focal point for examining how external pressures can destroy individual consciousness. The album suggests that modern industrial society creates conditions that systematically undermine mental stability. The work ultimately questions whether artistic success and psychological well-being are fundamentally incompatible, presenting mental deterioration as both a personal tragedy and a broader cultural phenomenon reflecting societal dysfunction.

Mutual Ambivalence

I suggest that the sense of *ambivalence* of the maturing boy can be related not only to *Oedipal disillusionment*, as Freud suggested, but also to the father's own disposition. Without attempting to make a universal claim, as Freud did, I would suggest that it is possible at times to examine the boy's ambivalence as an emotional response, *reaction formation*, to some failure on the father's side to maintain the same loving position he held towards the boy in the past. André Green (1927–2012) first referred to such a process when coining the term the *Dead Mother*. Green's idea of the *dead mother* describes what happens when a mother becomes emotionally unavailable to her child, often because of her own grief, depression, or trauma. The child experiences her physically alive but emotionally dead. For the child, this is deeply confusing and painful because the mother is present but cannot respond with warmth or love. To cope, the child may shut down feelings, withdraw, or become overly self-reliant. Later in life, this pattern can affect relationships, making it hard to connect, trust, or feel fully alive with others, since early love felt lost but was never mourned.

While Green refers to the process as occurring in the very early days of the infant's development, I extend the term to refer to what happens to the boy's development in relation to the father's absence in adolescence. Such an absence is not necessarily a result of the father deliberately distancing himself from the boy but quite often a result of some event, external or internal, which emotionally over-engages the father, rendering him *emotionally absent* to the boy. That emotional absence remains mysterious to the boy and becomes a source of his disappointment once realizing that his pre-adolescent loving father has now changed and become preoccupied and distant.

When the father is emotionally absent but present physically, the boy's experiences are *uncanny*, as the father is both there and not there, alive and dead. Such an absence might be interpreted by the boy as a reaction to his own developmentally natural wish to relocate himself in relation to the father, a retaliation. This is experienced as an attack, *reaction formation*, and introduces *toxicity* to the relationship. That toxicity might be there as a natural product of the boy trying to assert himself, but when it corresponds with an actual emotional absence it can become too much for the boy to bear.

Such a toxic presence of the father at this developmental stage collides with the natural fantasy the child must overcome and even get rid of the father, as part of the oedipal process. The proverb *be careful what you wish for* resonates here. The boy's experience of the emotional absence of his father is tragically attributed to his own ambivalence. The boy is unable to see that the change his father underwent is due to external circumstances and not as a result of his fantasy.

The ensuing guilt creates a wound in the boy's mind. As I will elaborate later, Gil's ability to find solace in musical cultural objects as a container for his unconscious drama helped him to stay relatively intact and prevented an *emotional breakdown*. His ability to creatively find such an alternative was based upon his natural desire for the survival of the father as part of his desire to be reassured of the integrity of the world as a safe place.

And yet, it is important not to underplay the power of the ambivalent wish and the impact that its fulfilment might create. If at first there seems to be some integration between wishing to overcome the father and wishing his survival, one need only to refer back to Freud's (1939) acknowledgement that aggression was not the most dominant feature of the father and son relationship during adolescence. In *Moses and Monotheism*, he argued that even cannibalism might have had a holding function when the tribal individuals hated and feared their father as well as honoured him as a model and wished literally to take his place and digest him. The cannibalistic act is an attempt to ensure identification with the father by incorporating a piece of him.

The boy's ability to integrate those aspects and to survive such powerful forces of destruction allow him to repair his injured father's imago and continue with the developmental task of relocating himself in relation to his internal objects.

Sometimes this inner work cannot happen. When that is the case, the boy will feel less able to contain his mixed emotions. He will lose access to the space where he can process and transform these feelings and express them openly, and instead they will turn inward. Because he cannot digest them, these painful emotions will have to be pushed out in some way, otherwise they remain inside like a toxic presence that must be released. This release might show up as a symptom or, more hopefully, through a creative outlet. It is this last possibility that I want to explore further, especially through music and how teenagers identify with popular musical themes.

Listening to Music as Dreams

I suggest that some adolescents' interest in particular items of literature and music can be attributed to such creative use. In such a case, a careful interpretation of that specific piece of music or writing can contribute greatly towards the understanding of the boy's inner world.

The process of interpreting pieces of art, music, and literature is a part of the way in which we enrich our lives, imbuing those works with parts of ourselves so that we can feel nourished and represented by them. We add something to what we hear, and in that way transform it. We are not just making echoes but offer authentic response.

The work we do with pieces of culture we identify with, as my client Gil did as a boy with *Wish You Were Here* and *Tommy*, is comparable to the work we do with *dreams*. Dreams are not simply clues as to what we have repressed but contribute to the way our mind is formed. The way Gil related to the text and music was similar to the way one deals with dreams. In both instances, they served him both as sources of inspiration and solace but also formed part of his maturational process.

Dreams of course are no longer thought of as just disguised expression of repressed impulses, desires, and fears. Dreams and objects of culture allow for unconscious communication to enrich our lives. We engage in symbolic interpretation of a dream or a song and find their relevance to our lives. As this fictional study will demonstrate, when Gil was 13 years old, he listened to music and dreamt. His engagement with these contents allowed him to deal with his sense of fear and loss due to this reaction to his father's emotional absence and to develop himself around those experiences. He was engaged in a creative and playful activity through the music, which saved his life.

Gil was 34 years old when he sought therapy with me in my private practice, after ending a painful relationship with a woman with whom he had lived for four years. Though he was the instigator of their break-up and at first felt relieved to be on his own again, several weeks later he began experiencing sleep loss, poor concentration at work, moodiness, and irritability. He felt as if he was grieving over a beloved person without knowing who it was. He was, in his own words, *"experiencing bereavement without anyone actually dying around me!"*

Despite his depressive symptoms, he did his best to engage in understanding what was happening with him. He brought recollections of dreams to therapy, and his associations were abundant. My initial liking for him deepened, and I experienced myself in the transference as a loving father, appreciating the emergence of his personality. At times I felt slightly concerned, as a father would, when he reported episodes of deep despair which he dealt with by staying home, smoking weed, and listening to music until he fell asleep. It was a bit strange as we were in fact very similar in age, and I assumed that something else was also going on on that level.

The therapy was on its third month when the Jewish Holidays period came near. It meant that we would miss three sessions. All our efforts to find alternative dates were to no avail as we were both travelling abroad during the holidays. I noticed that he was disappointed but rebuked my efforts to put it out in the open.

When we returned from our respective holidays, he seemed more anxious. While on holiday abroad, he met a young woman with whom he started an intense affair. The affair continued after they returned but seemed to fill Gil with anxiety lest he again find himself stuck in a relationship he did not really want.

Towards the end of the session following his return, after a silence that lasted longer than usual, I noticed that he was humming quietly to himself. It was an almost indiscernible hum but loud enough so I could hear it without being able to recognize the tune. I let it pass that time and made a mental note to myself. It felt as if Gil was creating a private space within himself and within the process, in response to something that had been going on. At that point I remained in the dark and felt excluded from a part of the process, which impressed me as significant.

During the following session, the humming returned. I maintained my position of not commenting on it but also recognized that my abstinence was building up tension within me. It felt somewhat disproportionate to the event, and I wondered what the underlying unconscious communication being acted out between us was. I noticed that my preoccupation with the significance of the humming was interfering with my ability to pay close attention to Gil when he was speaking. I felt myself withdrawing from him and becoming somewhat absent as a retaliatory response to his distance from me.

The content of these two sessions centred on his dissatisfaction with the prolonged holiday affair. He related his reluctance to end it to the unfinished business with the relationship that had brought him into therapy initially. After some time, he paused, hummed, fell into silence, and then commenced to tell me a dream.

In his dream he was watching over his younger brother while his parents were going out. His father was dressed in clothes which seemed inappropriate, and he was unshaven and seemed distracted. His mother seemed oblivious. He watched them as they went out the door, and when he looked back at his young brother, he was gone. At that point Gil woke up. He said that he felt no fear though he knew he should have. Silence followed, and before I had a chance to say anything, he began humming, this time a different tune. Gil noticed my interest and asked with a smile if I recognized the tunes he had been humming.

I replied that it sounded familiar. I then repeated what I thought I heard him hum: *"It's a Boy, Mrs. Walker, it's a Boy! It's a Boy, Mrs. Walker, it's a Boy!"*, the theme song from The Who's *Tommy.*

Gil glowed in response to my recognition. He did not expect me to know that piece of music. He added that that was indeed the tune he had just hummed, but the previous one was different. It was Pink Floyd's theme from *Wish You Were Here.* It was a moment of closeness and understanding in the process which symbolized the *therapeutic alliance* that had formed between us.

The Absent Father

Gil was 15 years old when his father was called to service. Up until that moment, the family's life in 1970s' Tel Aviv could be characterized as comfortable middle class. Both parents worked, and Gil was doing well at school. Gil was the eldest child. His parents were loving towards the children and to one another. Gil shared his father's interest in football and went to Saturday matches with him. As a young man, Gil's father dreamt of becoming a professional footballer and showed promise. He played in a professional club, but a severe injury, which nearly crippled him at the age of 19, ended those aspirations.

The day Gil's father was called to service, 6th October, 1973, had been intended as a day when they would go to play together in the park. It was the beginning of the Yom Kippur War, when Israel was surprised by a joint and coordinated attack by Egypt in the South and Syria from the north. The Arabs chose that particular day, Yom Kippur, the Day of Atonement, as it is the most sacred day in the Jewish calendar, when many Jews, even if they are not particularly religious, fast and abstain from all activity. In retrospect, the attack on Israel on 7th October, 2023 was similarly a surprise (more of that in Chapter Eleven).

When his father came back after several weeks, which he had spent inside a tank on the Golan Heights in the north, Gil waited for him wearing the same outfit he wore the Saturday he had left, holding in his hands their football as a welcome-home gift. His father hardly smiled. His unshaven cheeks were withdrawn. He avoided his family and after a few minutes went into the bedroom and slept through the following 24 hours. Gil was devastated and could hardly be consoled by his mother. His disappointment soon turned into rage, which he only ended with sleep.

The memory of that return haunted Gil for years. Even though his father seemed much better the following day and dutifully took Gil to play football in the park that afternoon, Gil felt that his heart was not in it. He played with him like a robot and soon got tired and took Gil back home. They never played football again together after that afternoon. Gil gradually lost interest in football; he began to despise it and deride anyone who showed interest in the sport. They did not go to football matches the following season to support their favourite team, Maccabi Tel Aviv, and he once called his father "a moron" for trying to coax him into going to see a match together.

After his initial few days at home, his father went back to his work as an engineer but quite often took sick leave. Gil could not remember all the details but recalled that his father wasn't well for a few months.

Later, his experience of his father was still of a weak and fragmented figure, even though he seemed to have recovered. He was unable to articulate his wish for a more robust and stable father. He used the *Tommy* theme, another boy who had seemingly lost his father in war, to relate to a memory fragment of a boy who had lost his father and as a result lost his own competence in the world, escaping into fantasy.

During the following sessions, we tried to retrace the significance of the words uttered by the midwife who delivers the baby Tommy in the opening lines of the rock opera, as this had puzzled Gil for a long time. All he knew was that whenever he began listening to that album, which he did many times, he was seized with a deep sense of loss and longing.

In time, it became clearer that his adolescent preoccupation with the music, the lyrics, the narrative, and the cultural background of the fictional character of Tommy may have presented Gil with an opportunity to register, digest, and work through the emotional change he had experienced in the relationship with his traumatized but formerly beloved father.

While the music lacked conscious links with his own life experience, he continued to regard it as his own. It remained an object he was absorbed with, which gave him some degree of emotional and spiritual solace but failed to help him come to terms with the mundane physical reality of living with a traumatized father and the disturbed family which they had become.

In time, Gil began to recall more in the sessions, and he was also able to ask his father and mother about that traumatic time. His father was reticent at first, and his mother was surprised that it had affected him so strongly. She recalled that they had gifted Gil the LP as a present. It was only a month later that the 1973 war broke out, and his father was called to duty. The sounds of *Wish You Were Here* and *Tommy* were the soundtrack of those days for Gil, but he disassociated the memory of the music from the actual events of those months.

The memories from those days were scant. He knew that many of his father's friends were killed or injured during the early battles on the Golan Heights. Much later he learnt of the heroic battles that his father was part of. Even after his father seemed to have recovered, Gil remained particularly sensitive to the change in his father's inner state. Gil was left with a feeling that his father was not the same person in ways he could not even formulate himself. A gap was created, and that gap was filled with Pink Floyd's *Wish*

You Were Here and The Who's *Tommy*. His relationship with the music attempted to bridge over the tear that was created by his father's *emotional absence*. Listening to the blind, deaf, and dumb Tommy became a substitute. In a similar way, learning of the background for the creation of *Wish You Were Here* – i.e. Syd Barrett's mental breakdown – allowed him to dwell on these issues without realizing they had to do with his own fears.

He felt deprived of his senses by the traumatic transformation. He was shocked into a different defensive state when his father returned. In the rock opera, Tommy's father is killed in a fight with his mother's lover, whom Tommy came to recognize as a father figure. Syd Barrett's mind was shattered for reasons Gil could not yet understand but sensed were significant. Gil's father's life was indeed spared, but he was no longer the same man.

The break in the therapy opened that old wound. It led to a regression and the use of the music from *Tommy* and *Wish You Were Here* was again used as nonverbal compensation. Understanding that allowed Gil to reconnect his memories from that period. During the following sessions, Gil was able to work through the various aspects of his developmental *ambivalence* towards his father, which was brutally disrupted by his emotional absence. He was beginning to string the pieces together.

Emotional Absence

The music of *Tommy* and *Wish You Were Here* helped young Gil to deal with a pain he could not comprehend nor articulate verbally. It came to represent for him an effort to come to terms with an incomprehensible piece of reality. Its significance only became clear during the therapy, when it surfaced as a reaction to my absence.

Though the absence was seemingly mundane and anticipated, it evoked a deep reaction, as he unconsciously relived an earlier undigested experience. That experience contained a disassociated memory of Gil's father's *emotional absence*, which had never been properly understood by the boy. It has sunk into near oblivion, wrapped up in the music that was significant for Gil at that time.

What brought back the memory into consciousness, thus allowing its working-through in therapy, was the piece of music itself, hummed by Gil. Once the memory, with its previously disassociated feelings, was relived, Gil was able to come to terms with aspects of his relationship with his father. The father imago, which had been injured due to the father's emotional absence, was acknowledged more fully. This allowed Gil to let go and continue the delayed but natural process of separation from the beloved father-son paradigm. Consequently, Gil was able to deal more effectively with current relationships in his life. He was able to disengage the ambivalence he had felt towards his father during his adolescence from the sense of loss he had felt earlier.

Gil's father re-integration into his life after the war did not totally lead him to overcome the sense of injury. It remained unthought *known*, but thanks to Gil's embracing of *Tommy*, he was able to find a source of solace in his attachment to the music and its associated themes. This provided him with a transitional cultural object with which he could identify and onto which he was able to transfer his attachment.

Freud's Father

As a conclusion, I go back to interpret an instance in Freud's own relationship with his father, Jacob Freud (1815–1896). This incident will help, I believe, to further illustrate the way I understand Freud's 1914 essay, *Some Reflections on Schoolboy Psychology*, which served as the basis for this study.

This is not a reductionist attempt to link Freud's biography with the theoretical framework I used in this chapter. I use it as a suggestion of yet another example of the emotional ambivalence Freud refers to.

Freud recounts that when he was 10 or 12 years old, his father began to take him along on his walks and discuss various world issues. One day, to show how radically life had improved for Austrian Jews, Jacob Freud told his son a story. When he was a young fellow, one Saturday he went for a walk with a new fur cap on his head. He came across a local lad, who knocked off his cap into the muck with one blow and shouted: *"get off the sidewalk, you Jew"*. Young Sigmund asked his father what he did and was taken aback to learn that Jacob stepped into the road and picked up his cap rather than confront the antisemite. Jacob's submissive response did not seem heroic to young Sigmund and made his realize that his father was not a big, strong man.

Freud's realization that his father was not the omnipotent figure he had thought him to be helped him to form his ideas of the father imago. His disappointment stemmed from a case of *emotional absence* due to an external event which preoccupied the father's awareness to the extent that he was temporarily unavailable for the boy's projections. Freud viewed his father as absent not because of a physical disappearance but through his reluctance to stand up to antisemitic verbal abuse, which functioned as what Freud the son viewed as a weakness. The racial abuse his father tolerated without an apt response created a sense of abandonment in the young Freud. In a sense, one could argue that Freud was left alone in a hostile Gentile environment without the benevolent protection of his father, both as a real presence but even more significantly as an injured and partially absent *father imago*.

Freud's connection to Jacob can be seen in the letter he wrote to Wilhelm Fliess after his father's death in 1896 to attest his attachment to him as well as deal with some unresolved issues. Freud seems surprised by his own pain when he writes that without knowing how and why the death of his father has affected him deeply. He then makes a surprising statement which seems to go way beyond a description of the illness which caused his father's death when he adds that his life was over a long time before he died.

Freud refers here to the death or at least the decline of the father imago he had experienced during his early adolescence. The disappointment he experienced from his father in his response to the antisemitic abuse, and probably other events which remained unreported, were felt deeply.

It is not only his father that was injured but Freud's own sense of belonging. The injury to the father imago, which was left unattended, resulted in an injury to his sense of belonging. One must also remember that it was after his father's death in 1896 that Freud began his *self-analysis*, which laid the foundation for the writing of his work on dreams, published in 1900. It was the father's absence which motivated Freud to undergo the inner quest which gave birth to psychoanalysis.

Joining the dots and drawing parallels between Freud's, Gil's, and Pink Floyd's *Wish You Were Here* and The Who's *Tommy* stories is maybe stretching the analogy a bit too far. I will conclude this chapter with a slight tongue-in-cheek question.

It is curious that in the rock opera Tommy becomes a messianic figure for a while until he can rework his grief. Was Freud too in danger of becoming a Messiah, against his own will, on account of some of his followers advocating too strict adherence to his creative theories?

It is left for us, who are inspired critically by his ideas, to continue the vigorous study of the self so as not to be turned blind, deaf, and dumb by ignorance and superstition.

Chapter 8

Echoes Across Generations

Psychoanalysis, War Trauma, and Post-Memory in Israel

In this chapter, the last one in this book that describes clinical work, I will use four *interdisciplinary concepts* which I have found over the years to be central to my clinical work. I will apply them to the fictional study of Vered, a young Israeli woman, who turned to therapy due to an anxiety attack during her obligatory Israeli Defense Forces (IDF) military service. Almost all Israeli citizens are conscripted to a two- to three-year army service when they turn 18, men and women alike. A lot of them continue to do reserve service after they complete their obligatory service. Many of them pay with their lives. Their families and the communities they live in also pay a heavy price. The scope of this chapter does not allow for a full review or discussion of the subject, which also includes casualties within neighbouring countries. I will focus on symptoms exhibited by people who were involved in acts of war or terror, which are often exacerbated by previous life events. In Israel, such previous life events often relate to what happened to the parents and grandparents of those individuals during the Holocaust.

The Return of the Repressed, and Hermeneutics and Testimony

The *Return of the Repressed* is one of Freud's earliest ideas, which he first introduced in 1896 and repeated in his book on dreams, later somewhat revising and developing it in one of his case studies, his letters, and finally in his work on repression in 1915.

What remains constant in his description is the statement that repressed material will always seek a conscious expression and that it is indestructible – i.e. it is never lost to oblivion but only hides from awareness until such a time occurs which prompts its emergence as a symptom, dream, or creative expression.

This is pertinent to this clinical illustration in the sense that it offers one possible interpretation to the question as to how events in the client's childhood, which at the time seemed unrelated to her direct sensory experience (and therefore minor in their impact), have left such a strong and potent trace as to contribute to her present-day predilection. The repressed but intact contents of undigested and perhaps indigestible mental content were only able

DOI: 10.4324/9781003683162-8

to return and re-appear through dreams as well as disturbing symptoms and creative expressions.

The second key concept, *the Hermeneutics of Language*, bridges the gap between literature and psychoanalysis. Language is not simply a medium for the expression of the self; it is integral to the creation of the self. In the therapeutic setting, with its focus on talking as the principal means of communication, narrative and language are among the main ways in which individuals bring themselves into being.

This is particularly relevant to listening with the utmost attention to the complexities of the human voice of the client. The onus of this attention is placed upon the therapist, who must master a very complex attention span which stretches like a web almost infinitely. In Chapter One, I introduced Akhtar's model of listening, which is still an inspiration.

The focus is of course the narrative of the client. But the narrative is never one dimensional and is refracted by the particular cultural tone which the therapist has to recognize and become familiar with. This may be true to all cultures, but working in Israel, the therapist has to differentiate between not only several nationalities but also widely differing ethnic backgrounds, places of residence, and varying degrees of religiosity.

Another dimension would be the subtleties of the client's narratives as they alter from one session to another and within each session in relation to their emotional state and transference position. Interlinked with this last dimension is the therapist's own multi-layered narrative. The links between the two narratives create yet another dimension which extends the web of attention deep into the unconscious realm, where both voices form a new and yet-undiscovered territory.

The exploration of this unknown territory needs to be studied with the same minute and careful approaches that one adopts when reading a literary text which contains unfamiliar vocabulary and syntax. Thus, the therapist listens to the client's words, and his own, as to a text being written during the session. This text is a live event, linked to past occurrences. It is a dance of minds where the client's whole being interacts, consciously and unconsciously, with the therapist's. The text analysed, therefore, is not only what the therapist or the client says but the whole web, or matrix, that evolves during their time together. And in this web are caught words, images, memories, objects, and introjects.

The third key concept refers to Dori Laub's work on *testimony* in history and psychoanalysis. Laub (1937–2018), himself a Holocaust survivor and psychoanalyst who worked with Holocaust survivors, writes about the attention that is required of the listener in the cases of trauma. He states that whoever listens to the story of extreme human suffering requires themselves to deal with an unprecedented situation. By listening to the story of the survivor, the listener is acting both as a witness to the story itself and, perhaps more importantly, to the feelings associated with it, belonging both to the listener and the survivor. What they listen to most, at least initially, is the experience of the *absence of language* in the trauma.

The story, as it has not been told until then, is a mental gap. Without a human *witness*, it does not exist in tangible human and verbal dimensions and therefore acts as a force of nature, as a storm does. The listener is a participant in the traumatic event and is a partner in creating the emotional and cognitive space required for its verbal witnessing. In order to not let the forces of the trauma (the storm) transform the listener into being a survivor himself, they need to be able to remain somewhat separate.

Laub suggests that this position is attained by two paths: the first is a prior knowledge by the listener of the territory into which they are travelling and the second is their own ability to bear witness to their own process. Thus, the therapist who wishes to create a therapeutic environment which will facilitate the witnessing of an untold trauma needs to sharpen their listening so that they can become attuned both to the multiplicity and diversity of the client's narrative, conscious and unconscious, as well as to their own passage through the client's tale.

Post-Memory

The fourth and perhaps hardest to comprehend concept is the idea of *post-memory*. Post-Memory describes a significant event that happened before one's birth and has been passed on through multi-generational transmission to one's unconsciousness in such a way as to shape a part of it. It becomes a part of one's own narrative but is not quite conscious and shows itself through various indirect forms such as particular symptoms. An example would be various uncanny phenomenon whereby one cries at certain films, feels anxious at other times, and is avoidant of familiar events without being able to understand the reason.

When does a post-memory come into existence? There must be some external stimulus in the shape of an artefact, whether a photograph, letter, film, or even a remembrance of a story once told. This stimulus evokes a sense of a forgotten memory which cannot be accessed but carries a strong emotion. Trying to gain more data concerning that memory begins the process of bearing a testimony. If successful, this kind of remembrance, not unlike archaeological digging, reveals links formed between that external stimulus and recollections of family stories which echo someone else's experience. A web of relations and association, a matrix of meanings and possibilities, is created, sending the individual in search of more clues.

This is not an ordinary search that one can easily abandon if it does not immediately yield satisfactory results. Rather, it is an obsessive search that becomes a goal in itself, leaving its subject matter somewhat in the shadow. A search that outsiders view with a slight worry, lest you dedicate unreasonable amounts of time, emotional and mental energy, and sometimes even considerable resources to it; a search that ultimately consumes you.

I am including this rather baffling concept on the basis of the work I have done myself with my own post-memory when studying the history of my maternal grandmother. Having had the fortune of being in possession of hundreds of letters and other items exchanged between three branches of the family in Paris, Tel Aviv and Thessaloniki during World War II, I was able to form a narrative around a haunting experience I had for years. I was lucky at that time to meet with Holocaust scholars who introduced me to the concept of post-memory, which served as the framework for my study, later published by Routledge.

In the following fictional case study, I will illustrate how these concepts come to play as an example of the special attention psychotherapists need to pay to stories which have not yet been told.

Being a Female Paratrooper

Vered was 24 years old when she was called up for her three-week reserve force assignment as a paratrooper in an elite unit of the IDF. At that time, she was still single though fairly active socially and quite pleased with the way her life was going. She was in her second year at university studying law, which pleased her family but was considered by her only as a stepping stone towards a professional future she was not yet sure about.

Vered was referred to me by a psychiatrist in the IDF with whom I had worked in the past. He thought that Vered needed to see a civilian therapist who was familiar with current military mental health practices in the army, as I was.

The Mental Health Department in the IDF has grown both numerically and qualitatively over the last few decades and in particular after the first Lebanon war in the early 1980s. The scope of this chapter does not permit expanding further on this point, but it is significant to affirm that soldiers suffering from trauma and other mental disorders caused by and/or appearing during their military service are taken more seriously than in the past and treated accordingly.

When Vered made the first contact with me it was by email. The email arrived with nothing appearing in the subject heading, and its content was very brief. She wrote that Dr. Litvak, the military psychiatrist, had given her my number. When she did ring, a few hours later, she wanted to make an appointment straight away, as if the email brief exchange had established enough contact. I sensed that she was delaying and perhaps avoiding contact but doing so in an elaborate and confusing way.

The association which I found myself contemplating after hanging up was that she had to prepare me for seeing her, and this she chose to do by employing a variety of communication methods, as if to make doubly sure that I could be reached. A slight sensation of being toyed with and perhaps even manipulated lingered on and evoked a mixed sense of curiosity and slight dread about our first session.

When meeting her for the first time, I was very aware of the fact that it was not *without memory and without desire*, as Wilfred Bion advocated. When Vered entered the room, the atmosphere that surrounded her was in stark contrast to all that I have described above. She seemed calm and collected, spoke with fluency and self-confidence, and related her complaint in a very leisurely manner. I felt ill at ease with my own pre-conceived judgement and almost paralyzed by the sense that I had been wrong in my initial assessment.

She told me that the last time she was called up for military service the small unit she was part of ran into some trouble in one of the West Bank refugee camps. During a routine patrol, stones were thrown at the armoured vehicle that they were driving in. One of the soldiers spotted a group of youngsters standing nearby who he thought were responsible, and the driver of the vehicle made an abrupt turn and sped forward in such a way which caused the vehicle to run down three of the youngsters.

When other Palestinians who were in the area noticed that, hell broke loose. It was only a couple of hours later that they were able to pull out of the camp, aided by other armoured vehicles that were called in. During that time, once she had realized that they had run over the youngsters, she felt paralyzed and sat in the corner of the vehicle almost without being able to participate in the actions. Her fellow soldiers of course noticed her predicament but were too busy dealing with the situation themselves to do anything about it. Upon returning to base and following a briefing, she was immediately referred to the military psychiatrist, who then referred her to me after a few consultation sessions.

The story was indeed a harrowing story, and yet she told it as if she was reporting something that happened to someone else. I thought to myself *that a dissociative defence mechanism* was playing a part in the clinical picture to allow her to be so calm and so cut off from the content of her story. She carried on saying that since that event she was in fact in serious doubt as to whether she would ever want to go back to serve in the IDF.

She then said that she thought that her reaction at the time was an expression of something she had felt deeply a long time ago. She had always considered herself dovish as far as Israeli politics were concerned. Serving as part of the elite military unit as she did was justified by her as what all people of her age must do. After that incident, which she thought was the fault of the driver of the armoured vehicle, she was no longer able to justify being part of military actions whose sole purpose seemed to be to police and oppress the occupied Palestinian population. What she wanted from me, she said, was not so much therapeutic help but help in getting her off the register so that she could be dismissed from further military service.

Working with Dreams: The White Hotel

At that point, my heart sank. Not so much because I thought that dismissing Vered from further military service was a bad idea but because I was afraid that her retreat into a concrete solution, which was based upon even heavier repression, was a sad move. As she was not the first soldier I have treated in such circumstances, I thought of suggesting that we meet a few times for me to be able to assess her condition and see how I could respond to her request. She agreed but wanted me to know that even if I did not provide her with the necessary documentation, she would nevertheless refuse to go back to military service, even if it meant going to jail.

All this took place in early 1996, a few months after the assassination of the Israeli PM, Mr. Yitzhak Rabin (1922–1995), by a Jewish right-wing terrorist. Again, the scope of this chapter does not allow for much further elaboration, but it is important to mention that the public atmosphere was laden with strong emotions, ranging from rage to deep mourning, following the actual assassination and its obvious *Oedipal and patricide implications* for Israeli society, regardless of one's political leanings.

Vered had been raised by her parents in a loving and attentive way. Though both parents were busy professionals, they had been able to manipulate their work schedules so that Vered and her older sister were always in their focus. They also had substantial support from their grandparents, who were still active. Vered felt lucky to have them around when she was a child. In particular, she enjoyed the company of her paternal grandmother, whom she described as an eccentric but loving character. She said that most people found it hard to be around her as she was too direct and confrontational, but her grandmother spent many hours telling her tales of her early childhood in Slovakia. It was a happy childhood in Germany which was cruelly disturbed by the rise of the Nazi regime.

Six months into therapy, Vered brought me her first dream.

Dream work is a key element in my concept and practice of psychoanalytic psychotherapy. I invite dreams both from my clients and from myself just as I invite other unconscious communication. Working with dreams means using both symbolic interpretations and relying upon *dream-work* to do its silent job of elaborating and constructing aspects of the multi-layered self. Thus, the ensuing dialogue about the contents of the dreams and the arising associations, both by the client and by me, are primarily about weaving a web of connotations and meanings which facilitate and enable the transformative thrust of the therapeutic process.

In Vered's dream, she was flying or falling from a great height, above the earth's atmosphere but also from the 8th floor of her parents' house. The fall took a long time, and she wondered when she would hit the ground. At the same time, she was also down below on the ground, preparing the surface for her eventual fall. She tried to make the ground soft. While falling, she passed through the clouds and felt relieved because it meant the fall would soon be over. It seemed that the clouds were also softening the forthcoming crash by slowing her down. She reached the ground, and it was soft, like sand. Her parents had been observing her the whole time but were indifferent to her plight. She rolled on to the ground and then got up, unharmed.

The dream was recounted in an excited manner, revealing that something important was being communicated, though what it was she did not know. She just felt that it was an important dream. I waited for her to bring up more associations, but she remained silent and looked at me with expectation.

I had an idea or two in relation to the content but first applied my attention to interpreting her silence. I suggested that the speed with which she wanted me to resolve the dream was akin to the speed with which she was falling in the dream. She grimaced but remained silent for a minute or so. Then she said she was disappointed. What I had said meant nothing.

I felt moved by a sense of helplessness which permeated the room. I commented upon this and said that it seemed that the dream, her emotional response to it and my words, had created a powerful situation here and now that we should try and understand. To my surprise, Vered conceded and said that I was probably right. But she remained quite sullen until the end of the session.

When Vered did turn up for the next session, she said that she only came back to tell me something. After leaving the previous week, something dawned on her. She realized that she was disappointed with the intervention about the dream because it reminded her that therapy was *"just words and words meant nothing in the real world"*. She then directed her gaze at me and said: *"Just as my grandmother always used to say. All the good words are useless. What's the point of talking when death is out there?"*

I began joining the dots. I knew by then that her parents did not get along. They had remained together, but in her teenage years she had noticed that in fact they hardly spoke to one another in general, let alone show any affection or warmth. Nor did they seem to argue or fight much. They were just together, being there with not much going on between them. She could not bear to be a witness to an emotional reality that needed to be witnessed by someone. What needed to be witnessed – the reality of her parents' relationship – was just too unbearable for her. She would leave the room and often went to visit her grandmother, who lived in the building next door.

She said that my interpretation of the dream reminded her that sometimes there is nothing you can say. This feeling corresponded to her position while crouching down inside the armoured vehicle while out there children were dead because of a careless move her comrade had made.

She then pointed to a particular book on my bookshelf, *The White Hotel*, by D.M. Thomas (1935–2023), and said:

> *Do you know this book? My grandmother let me read it when I used to hide in her apartment from my parents. I think she meant well, but that book destroyed me. It was in that book that I found out how pointless talking really was. Only actions matter. It does not matter what you say, only what you do and what other people do to you that matter. That's what my grandmother used to say. And she should know. She survived the worst of humankind.*

Clients referring to books in my library is something I have gotten used to over the years, and yet each time it happens I deal with it differently depending on the varying circumstances. The book in question was a fictional account of a psychoanalytic treatment of a client of Freud's and all that happened to her in and after the treatment. In the first half, the book describes in detail her treatment, focusing mainly on *the love transference* that transpired. The treatment was inconclusive. The client then marries a young Jewish opera singer. They have a child together and move to Kiev in 1920. The husband runs away, and she and her child are captured by the Nazis in 1941 and massacred in Babi Yar in September of that year.

Vered recounted its narrative to me and summed its impression upon her:

> *What's the point of all this psychoanalytic babble? At the end, after Freud treated her, she was killed by the Nazis! So, what good are all her insights? What does it matter that she understood how she was brought up this or that way? At the end she died of hunger by those animals! Psychotherapy is pointless when there's a war going on, and we are at war now and need to be at war forever so that they don't do this to us again.*

There was silence. Vered was upset in a way I had never seen her before. I had the feeling that it was not just her own words that she was speaking. I felt I was allowed to witness a part of her that was in conversation with her grandmother, the Holocaust survivor.

She described her grandmother, Edith, as the one person whom she could relate to in the family during her adolescence. She would sit in her kitchen, watch her cook, and listen to her stories about times past. Some of those stories were very pleasant stories and described the lifestyle she and her family enjoyed in pre-Holocaust Europe. But quite often, a bitter note creeped into her story, and she told of her struggles, her plight in the camps, and the many losses she suffered. She almost always made a point of ending those stories in such a way as to show her the greatness of the Jewish people that survived the Holocaust.

More than once, she was left with a horror she could hardly digest. It was then she felt paralyzed, contemplating what she could not witness, trying to think and picture what could not be pictured.

Vered went silent. She looked down at the carpet and then looked up at me and said:

> *You know, you were right, it was like that in the armoured vehicle. I was sitting there on the floor, knowing we have just killed innocent civilians, and I felt I could do nothing. It was the same feeling of horror. I was a witness to something I did not want, did not need, to be a witness to. I only wish I could erase it from my mind. I only wish I could go back to a time when all this did not happen. But I can't. It keeps coming back, again and again.*

This is Not My Memory!

In time, she was able to see how her parents' quarrels and slight neglect pushed her to spend more time with her grandmother. Her influence was massive, but there was a price to pay. She served as Vered's haven, but within that haven she was exposed to tales of a world that frightened her. Hearing her mourn her dead relatives and hearing her tell of her time in the concentration camps and her survival filled her with admiration and horror. But mostly it filled her with a sense of helplessness. That sense had become lodged within her as an entity that felt suffocating, one she could not expel.

Vered felt that trying to get rid of that would amount to a betrayal of an integral part of her being. She had to keep it inside. It felt like a memory which did not belong to her but which she had formed a strong attachment to. During the following sessions, she recalled more and tried to understand.

The work I have done myself on my own family's survival of the Holocaust enabled me to understand emphatically Vered's discovery of her *post-memory.* I had one too. She had also come by some of the material I have published, and we were able to share grandmother stories …

Vered's therapy lasted four years. The brief segment described was part of a journey that stretched along a circuitous path, trailing signposts of the past and present. It was a journey into the mind of one Israeli citizen and soldier who suffered what would have been described in the past as *shell shock* but which turned out to be the impact of a cluster of injurious events.

During the third year of the treatment, her grandmother died. She was fortunate enough to have been able to spend meaningful time in her presence almost up to her death. Having realized the ambivalent impact she had had upon her as an adolescent, she was able to both listen to her in a way which comforted her and remain at a safe distance. She no longer felt like a trapped soldier sitting defenceless inside an armoured vehicle, fearing to witness what was going on in the outside world.

She no longer sought to be dismissed from military service. She did ask to be transferred to another unit so that she would be less exposed to such actions. It seemed like a reasonable solution to an insoluble situation.

Postscript

It is not often that I have a chance to find out what has happened to a client after therapy is over. With Vered, I was lucky to glean a few details.

As I will describe in Chapter Eleven, I am a part of *The Road to Recovery* Israeli voluntary organization. It was established by Yuval Roth, whose brother was butchered by a Hamas terrorist attack in 1993. Rather than surrender to grief and revenge, Roth decided to dedicate his life to try and make a difference and established the organization which now is responsible for driving hundreds of Palestinian children and adults from the checkpoints around Israel to receive life-saving medical treatments in Israeli hospitals. They are driven there by hundreds of Israeli volunteers, who drive them in their private cars. Roth describes each such drive as a "little peace".

One day, I was pleased to see Vered in one of our volunteers meetings. I thought it was a good sign that she had seemingly regained her sense of agency in joining a social activity.

Chapter 9

The Psychoanalytic Geography of Exile

Home, Loss, and Creative Return

Creativity is one of the themes I study in this book. I see creativity as both an innate human drive as well as a capacity we can develop and expand, especially at times of inner or external distress and threat. I think of creativity in the broadest possible way. It is the capacity to engage with one's life circumstances in a way that enables you to feel like an active player rather than a submissive consumer of forces seemingly greater than yourself. Creativity relies on having *hope* in one's ability to act upon and transform one's existential circumstances, though as they might be.

Surely it has been noted that I almost always begin my explorations with reference to Freud. This is not because I believe his work holds all the answers or is always accurate. I do, however, happen to find his particular stamina and dedication very inspiring. Despite his many faults, not least his many misconceptions about women and the universal nature of his assumptions, I still have some reverence for his attempt to create a meta theory that would support both our clinical pursuits as well as our efforts to lead lives based upon greater awareness and reliance on rationality.

I therefore begin this chapter, a study of creativity and exile, the first of the last three chapters of this book which move away from purely clinical work, by reading his 1908 essay *Creative Writing and Day-dreaming*, where he outlines what he thinks enables an individual to become a creative writer. In this essay, he questions what such an individual possesses, or what possesses him, to enable engagement in the creative process. I hope to expand on this and show how creativity helps the individual to come to terms with their *secret wound.*

Freud suggests we should look for the first *traces* of imaginative activity in childhood when the child's primary and intense occupation is with *play.* He suggests that like the child the creative writer plays in creating a world of their own, assembling the things in their world in a new and creative form.

I will not attempt in this chapter to unravel the childhood origins of writers' creativity but rather conduct a study of the process through which three writers who have had a great influence on me sought to creatively form *a home* for themselves at times of stress by the act of writing.

DOI: 10.4324/9781003683162-9

By reading certain passages from the works of Lawrence Durrell, Sigmund Freud, and Aharon Appelfeld, I shall study the way the theme of their lost homes resonates in their writing, creating in their words that which had been lost by the circumstances of their lives.

Psychoanalysis and Literature

The relationship between literature and psychoanalysis has already been dealt with throughout this book, based on my belief that language as a vehicle for understanding human consciousness is a cornerstone of contemporary psychoanalytic theory. That is not to say that language is all, but it is certainly an avenue one must explore in the search for *authenticity*.

Literature and psychoanalysis are siblings and as such have a complex relationship, often competing for sovereignty to comprehend human consciousness. Literary interpretation offers a unique liminal space where biographical fact and fictional invention intermingle. At times, the biographical matrix of the author seems to overshadow the text; at others, the fictional universe appears to stand autonomously, detached from its creator's life. The most nuanced readings, however, arise from a subtle dialectic between the two, revealing that neither biographical nor fictional elements can be wholly extricated from the act of interpretation. Any assertion of biography as pure, unmediated truth overlooks the inherently constructed and imaginative nature of language itself, an ongoing creative act, often unconscious, always mediated.

In 1897, Freud conducted what is often considered the first psychoanalytic literary interpretation, analysing a text by the Swiss poet Conrad Ferdinand Meyer (1825–1898). Freud claimed to have uncovered a repressed memory concerning an incestuous liaison with the poet's sister, a revelation that fuelled his excitement over the psychoanalytic potential to illuminate hidden truths in literature and in therapy. Indeed, he would later suggest that literature, and poetry in particular, might access the deeper strata of the human mind than psychoanalysis itself. For Freud, the writer was one who successfully sublimated unconscious (often sexual) fantasies into coherent narratives without compromising mental equilibrium. Writing became a space where the imperfections of reality could be transformed and contained.

In this context, I propose to examine the themes of *home* and *leaving home*, as represented in the writings of Freud, Durrell, and Appelfeld, as such a symbol: layered, elusive, and richly interpretable.

In particular, I will explore the *uncanny* nature that characterizes the relationship to *home* in these works. Home, conventionally understood as a symbol of safety, continuity, and belonging, is revealed in these texts to be a destabilized and haunted concept, its promise of security irreversibly fractured.

As mentioned in Chapter One, the German term *das Unheimliche* (the uncanny) encapsulates this ambivalent experience. In his 1919 essay on the subject, Freud writes that *Heimlich* is an ambivalent and contrary word, meaning one thing and its opposite, *Unheimlich*. Drawing on E.T.A. Hoffmann's (1776–1822) gothic tale, Freud concludes that the uncanny is triggered when one becomes uncertain whether something is alive or dead, real or artificial. This disquieting feeling, he contends, originates in early infantile development: the child's unconscious fabrication of a double, a mental twin, to manage overwhelming experience. Though this *Doppelgänger* recedes with development, it leaves unconscious *traces*, which may resurface when we face ambiguity in our surroundings or within ourselves.

Home may be conceptualized not just as a stable physical location but as an emotional terrain, part interior, part lost, part remembered. To seek one's *home* is to embark upon a search for the self, a process that unfolds throughout life and culminates only in death. This inner journey often emerges in moments of rupture: personal crises, migrations, or sociopolitical upheaval. During such times, the implicit bond between the self and one's habitat, usually taken for granted, becomes fraught with fragility and ambivalence. These moments mark not only change, but loss, and everyone negotiates this loss in ways shaped by cultural, economic, and familial contingencies.

For the writer, such existential tremors may find expression in the act of writing. Writing thus becomes not merely an act of narration but a ritual of *mourning*, an instrument of emotional reconstruction. It creates a space for grief, reflection, and, ultimately, transformation. An example of this is the moment the familiar, *Heimlich*, becomes strange, *unheimlich*. The loss of the familiar makes space for hybridity, a fusion of old and new, a reconfiguration of meaning. This metamorphosis need not stem from catastrophe alone; it may arise from introspection, revelation, or the slow reconfiguration of memory.

Freud named this process *Nachträglichkeit*, a retroactive attribution of meaning whereby past experiences are revised and re-signified in light of the present. This phenomenon, central to psychoanalytic work, often unfolds in therapy and is mirrored in literature.

In this light, I suggest that Appelfeld's, Durrell's, and Freud's writings serve as acts of symbolic restitution: a home rebuilt not with bricks and mortar but with words and memory from a lost world and a mind shaped by displacement and survival. The three writers are indeed very different in many aspects. I hope that it is not only my interest in them that justifies bringing them together for this study. I shall begin by briefly recounting their histories and then proceed to a deeper and detailed analysis of some of their work.

Appelfeld was 9 years old when the Romanian army occupied his hometown, Jadova, Romania, in 1941, after a year under Soviet control. He was deported with his father after witnessing his mother's murder on the street. He spent the war years in a forced labour camp, escaped, and hid until the war's end before emigrating to Palestine, where he remained until his death in 2018.

Durrell was only twelve when sent by his father from his childhood paradise in India to a strict boarding school in England for *proper* British upbringing, as his father feared he would otherwise turn into a *wild man*.

Freud was forced to leave Vienna in 1938 at age 82 due to Nazi occupation and the growing danger to his well-being and life. With help from Marie Bonaparte, he moved to London with some family members, where he died a year later in 1939.

Leaving home – at any age, under any circumstances – is bound to be remembered. Under normal circumstances, it can be seen as a natural occurrence and part of the maturational process. Nevertheless, the circumstances under which it happens, and therefore its significance, vary dramatically. Each case needs to be investigated separately, bearing in mind that there will be no real similarities. This resonates with a very plain truth concerning therapy: no two individuals seeking help are the same, even if the circumstances and their characteristics seem very similar. Applied to the therapy of people who have been subjected to severe life events such as war, for instance, therapists often find that not all respond in the same way to same event. Some are traumatized while others are apparently not.

The Biblical proclamation that Abraham had to follow, *"Now the LORD had said unto Abram, Get thee out of thy country, and from thy kindred, and from thy father's house, unto a land that I will shew thee"* (Genesis 12:1), differs greatly from the 21st-century young man who leaves home for army or university. It differs markedly in the cases of 9-year-old Appelfeld, 11-year-old Durrell and 82-year-old Freud. Yet the symbolic quality of such events can be explored phenomenologically as forming a particular category defining the individual's sense of belonging to *a place called home.*

In the following pages, I will conduct a synchronic study of certain passages chosen from these three very different writers who nevertheless share, in my opinion, a very special and damaged connection to their homes as dealt with in their writing. It is not just a literary study. Rather it is a study of survival, which is what therapists deal with in their daily work. Reading the way Appelfeld, Durrell, and Freud relate their stories of survival is like listening to them in the therapy room. It is *bearing witness,* which is one of the most important functions that therapists carry, as I wrote in the Chapter One.

Appelfeld's Experience of Leaving Home

Aharon Appelfeld's words testify to his survival in his autobiographical book *The Story of a Life*, written in 1999, more than 50 years after he escaped Nazi-occupied Europe. He wrote that the book is not a summary but an attempt, perhaps a desperate attempt, to integrate the different parts of his life and convey them to the next generations. He adds that much has been lost and much corroded by oblivion. At first, it seemed that very little remained, yet when he laid one piece alongside another, he could see that not only had they been made whole by the years but they had even achieved some level of meaning.

Appelfeld was born 16th February, 1932, in Jadova, Romania (now Ukraine). He was an only child. When he was 9 years old, his mother was murdered before his eyes. He was then deported with his father to a forced labour camp, from which he escaped and managed to survive the war years. He emigrated to Palestine in 1946, settling there to become a world-renowned novelist.

A whole life in one paragraph. Each word contains details, emotions, loss. It is a life he explored through numerous novels and essays, making literature his life and his life literature. The home he had to leave is the place where memory and imagination dwell together.

The symbolism of the home and its derivatives is present throughout the book. Home is where he lived, a home he was forced to leave, and the text that grew out of writing about the memory of that home is where the author was now dwelling, a symbolic home.

For a home to be destroyed, abandoned, and then recreated through the act of writing, one needs first to establish that it was a home. When Appelfeld wrote *The Story of a Life*, he was already 67 years old. As he writes, the details of a childhood are subjected to the flow of time, and since memory is a living reservoir, listening to it and recording it is like listening to a dream, and like a dream, it shifts between reality and fantasy. Like a dream, memory is therefore a reservoir of unconscious details that can be revealed and understood through future interpretation.

Appelfeld writes that he has clear childhood memories of the time before the war broke, before he was 7 years old. He recalls family vacations in the Carpathian Mountains. The vastness, expanse, and beauty of those views soon diminished when the war broke out, and their lives were then crammed into a small room. The view of the world as a home was demolished when home became a narrow place, a temporary residence where life was spent mentally seeking a safe place that was never again found.

At what point can we say that Appelfeld lost his home? Was it at age 9, after his mother was murdered and he left his hometown with his father? Or perhaps it was earlier, at age 7, when the war began and brought devastating changes to him and his family? Or maybe it happened much later, when he started reflecting on his life through writing?

These questions may be impossible to answer. As he writes, once the war broke out, time became muddled and lost its normal sequence. Along with his sense of *home*, he also lost his sense of self as he had known himself before the war. What remained were his body sensations. His memory retreated into his body, recording his experiences through his physical being.

These kinds of responses are familiar to any therapist who works with people who have survived severe trauma and can only remember scant details of their past. The story they tell is often stored in their body, in their habits, sometimes destructive ones, that they developed to survive. The therapist's job is to decode these physical symptoms so the story can emerge into words, where it can be retold, connected to emotions, and woven into the survivor's life.

What was home for Appelfeld that was then lost? The first sense of belonging we can connect to home appears in Appelfeld's love for the view of the Carpathian Mountains. His descriptions of the mountains and rivers and the taste of strawberries show his deep connection to the world around him; he felt united with nature and its pleasures. He wrote that these sensations filled him with gentleness and tender care that he could still remember. These memories formed the core of his sense of belonging and shaped his essential self, staying with him through the difficult years. His identity was built around these sensory experiences.

I suggest that these pleasant sensory experiences that Appelfeld describes are actually *a screen memory*, a term Freud coined for memories that hide more complex truths underneath. His home, his world, was filled with the presence of the people he was about to lose. The house he grew up in, the house that was slowly becoming his true home, the sanctuary that fed his soul, was the home where his mother lived.

She appears in almost every memory. Whether they were walking in the countryside, preparing food, talking, or doing other activities around the house, she was always there. It is her presence, and young Appelfeld's loving gaze towards her, that transformed the house into a true home. She talked with him about God, she interrupted a band of travelling musicians when she thought their music might disturb him; she was always present, filling up his memory completely. She never left him alone for even a moment. Her closeness brought him such joy that even a brief separation made him feel sad.

But is it real? he wonders. Can he trust his memory when the images he recalls have become so unclear over time that they seem more like a dream? The sadness he describes when separated from his mother seems to predict the future. Soon, he would find himself drowning in that absence, overwhelmed by that sadness.

What came first? The sadness he remembers as a child before the war, an ordinary kind of childhood sadness, or is it the unbearable sadness that would later fill his world after he was forced to leave the home he loved so much, after losing his mother? Either way, that sadness filled the mind of the 67-year-old Appelfeld as he wrote his memoir.

Perhaps, then, Appelfeld never truly lost his home; he carried it within him all along. While the external markers of home, his mother, his town, his familiar world were violently stripped away, the deeper essence of *home* remained embedded in his body's memory and in his linguistic ability to recreate it in later years. His connection to the Carpathian landscape, the taste of strawberries, the feeling of merging with flowing water, these became his portable homeland. Through his writing, he was able to retrieve and honour this bodily archive of belonging, transforming trauma into art. In this way, his literature became both a search for home and the very act of coming home.

Describing a scene from a Shabbat at the local synagogue, where he felt both joy and confusion, he writes that he thought the people around him already knew how to speak to God, and only he was silent. He was filled with sadness at his inability to speak. Appelfeld's memories are soaked with the loss he would soon experience, and this loss is connected to losing his voice. The loss of speech is a common symptom among survivors of severe trauma. Often, people cannot talk for a long time about what they have lost. It is the patient listening of a therapist that gradually creates a safe space where they can find their voice again.

These memories are filtered through the awareness of the adult man who survived the disaster of losing his home. They can only be remembered through that lens of loss. He writes about his confusion as a 5-year-old child, standing outside his grandfather's synagogue and fearing its destruction. He looks at the synagogue, and what he sees is the sad future of his home. He remembers studying how the synagogue was built. The structure was so unstable that if it weren't for the ivy that wrapped around it and held it together, it probably couldn't stand on its own shaky foundation. He was gripped by a great unknown fear, a fear that at any moment people would come out of the building, grab him, and drag him inside. He describes the fear as being so real that he could actually feel the fingers of strangers pressing and poking at him.

What Appelfeld describes here matches the experience of the uncanny, when familiar things suddenly feel strange and threatening. The synagogue, which should be a familiar and safe place of worship and community, a home where he enjoyed spending time with his beloved grandfather and learning Jewish traditions, suddenly appeared to be falling apart and losing its strength. This is the heart of *the uncanny*: what seems alive is actually dead, what appears dead is actually alive. What seems safe is actually dangerous. The peaceful world that young Appelfeld thought surrounded his life was suddenly stripped away to reveal the cruel and life-threatening reality of losing one's home and safety.

What is the source of that great, unknown fear that Appelfeld describes? Appelfeld does not offer any direct explanation for why he was gripped with such fear at that moment or later. He remained haunted by it even when the family made their journey back home from visiting his grandfather. He writes that although he was pierced by an enormous sense of pain, he did not know how to talk about it.

I suggest that his sudden terror at the synagogue is actually the result of him sensing something familiar that had been buried in his mind and then reappeared in a strange form. The experience leaves him speechless. When he returns from the synagogue with his grandfather, he cannot talk. Only minutes later, when he is reunited with his mother, who had stayed behind to prepare the food, is he freed from his paralyzing fear.

At the synagogue, he faces something that only being with his mother can relieve. Is it the fear of the coming exile, the heart of which is his mother's death, that the 67-year-old Appelfeld returns to when writing his book? As speculative as this may seem, it becomes less so when we consider the deaths that will soon happen in his life: first his grandfather's death, then his mother's death. These losses inform and fill the remembering process that the 67-year-old author engages in while writing his memoir. What he returns to is death in retrospect, *Nachträglichkeit*.

This is a very clear description of the damage that *trauma* does to the mind of an individual. Trauma is caused when the individual is faced with an unexpected and serious threat to their lives. They are totally helpless and have no recourse to their survival instinct. They in fact experience death without actually dying. When that moment passes and they realize that they are alive after all, they are left with that inexplicable and incommunicable imprint of death upon their minds.

The loss of speech, the loss of language, is the near loss of life. Appelfeld wrote that it was only meeting with his mother, who understood his pain, who embraced him and drew him close to her, which allowed him back into life. While the origin of the fear seems to remain unknown at this stage, it is clear who can calm the young boy. Mother's comforting lap can soothe him to sleep with no words. At this stage, mother is the *witness* that sees his pain, recognizes his distress, and can reassure him.

That witnessing and soothing presence, so vital for mental health, is soon to be lost. In 1938 it became clear that they were trapped. Nothing went smoothly anymore. The safety, stability, and pleasure that has been associated with home is slowly changing. He recalls that people who had previously been welcome in their home, or who were trusted business partners or childhood friends, suddenly behaved as if they didn't know them or were transformed into enemies. People who were homely, familiar, and welcoming were slowly being transformed into an estranged, threatening, and frightening experience. Appelfeld quotes his grandfather, who said that the separation between the living and the dead is an illusion.

Death and the Disintegration of the Witness

The first victim is his father. Without yet knowing why, his father seems to the young boy to be sinking into a depressive mood. He recalls that after eating he'd sit on the sofa, his eyes closed, drowning within himself. Death hovered everywhere. He became withdrawn, spoke very little, and on his return from the exhausting attempts to get them transit papers, he would come straight into the kitchen, where mother would pour him a cup of coffee and spread two slices of bread with fruit preserves. He would eat distractedly and rapidly, finishing the two slices in an instant.

Only in retrospect does Appelfeld realize that those were the last days he was to spend at home. He cherished the memory of the few times his father was able to gather strength and stroll with him at night, as if saying goodbye to the beloved surroundings. The presence of his father slowly diminished. What maintained the sense of home, soon to be destroyed, was the constant presence of mother. She continued to act as the living spirit of the house.

The bad spirits persevered and deepened. The next victim was grandfather. His death in that summer was the one but final blow. It happened at the end of the summer, on a clear and cloudless day. Grandfather dozed off and never awoke from his sleep. The house had changed beyond recognition.

The disintegration of the home was gradual. There is no direct or elaborate description of the moment that house was left. There were several events that together cluster as signifying the symbolic and concrete process of *leaving home*: grandfather's death, father's depression, mother's despair. The move from the childhood house, the primeval home, into the Ghetto, is not elaborated upon. Such a transition was processed without words, as if the mind of the young boy was unable, unwilling, or not mature enough to symbolically register the process. There was a reason for the lack of clear mental memories. He wrote that the sense of things going on as if nothing had happened hurt him.

What was diminishing was mother's presence; she could witness and relate the events to the young boy. Without an adult containing the sense of bewilderment that he experienced and allowing a process of *mentalization*, it had sunk directly into the unconscious levels of his mind, showing its presence and register through his body.

His parents became silent. Even mother sat on the floor without uttering a syllable. The disintegration of mother as a witness whose presence could make sense of the insensible events, that could try to guide the young boy through those perilous days, was catastrophic.

Felman and Laub write about the immense significance that bearing witness and testifying to catastrophic events has. To bear witness is to maintain authenticity. It comes down to testifying before an audience of readers or future witnesses, and it is more than simply to report a fact or an event or to relate what has been lived, recorded, and remembered. Memory is conjured through the testimony essentially to address another individual, to communicate to a listener, to appeal to a community. To testify is to attempt to step into someone else's shoes, to relive their experience and preserve it in an emphatic and responsible way. Bearing witness forms a subjective narrative of the survival of the individual, omitting nothing. To testify is thus not merely to tell the story but to commit oneself, and to commit the narrative, to others: to take responsibility for the truth to be told, for something which, by definition, goes beyond the personal, in having validity and consequences.

Without such a testimony, young Appelfeld had to rely upon himself. He had to turn the testimony into his own body. He wrote that he had forgotten much, even things that were very close to him, places in particular, dates, and the names of people, and yet he could still *sense* those days in every part of his body. Memory has deep roots in his body. He testifies that he still hasn't found the right words to give voice to those intense scars in his memory.

I find Appelfeld's statement very pertinent to therapy. As I wrote at the beginning of the book, we are daily faced with experiences which defy clear verbal articulation. We sense what our clients tell us through *transference*, through *sensual experience*, and struggle to make those experiences conscious. We do that not simply to understand but to bring those deeply buried experiences to the surface so that the client can regain their sense of *agency*. Uncovering these experiences can be cathartic but not necessarily healing or easy to experience. If those experiences are uncovered, it still takes a lot of attention and care in the process of *working through* to try and mitigate the terrible pain that these experiences are entwinned with.

The final point signifying the collapse of home is an auditory one. His mother was murdered at the beginning of the war. He didn't see her die, but he did hear her one and only scream. With her death, home was destroyed as real concrete place where he could feel safe. But she did not disappear completely. She became a presence within. He felt her death deep inside him, but at the same time felt her alive within. He recalls that any time he is happy or sad, he sees her face.

Appelfeld's mother has become a representation of the uncanny. She is dead and yet alive. He sees her face even though she is dead. She becomes a symbol, a testimony, that the body remembers and brings up in times of excitement. In that sense, if mother is *home*, he has never left home. To affirm that, he keeps remembering having thought since he was a child that even though he knew she was dead he kept expecting her to return.

From the age of 7, young Appelfeld had to deal with an increasing sense of threat to the safety of his being and his home. It culminated catastrophically with the murder of his mother and his deportation, alongside the separation from his father not long after.

His story of survival is recounted in many of his books. As a boy, he was able to hide and live to tell his story. His ability to use language in the creative way that he did gave him a second chance. So many Holocaust survivors in Israel did not possess his gift of writing, and their stories remained untold for many years. They survived physically, raised families, often replacing the ones that were murdered, and formed the generation that helped the establishment of Israel. Emotionally, they often remained mute, transmitting the horrors of their survival to the next generations, as I have expanded upon in various parts of this book, especially in Chapter Eight.

Their lack of speech was not only a result of their inability to share their experiences. Often it was also because they felt that there was no one listening. In the early days of the state, many Holocaust survivors felt they would burden the young generations with their stories and thus impede the establishment of the new Jewish state. It was only during the 1970s that more and more survivors were able to tell their stories as there were more and more people ready to listen to them. Like in therapy, for a story to be told, to be witnessed, there needs to be *a live presence* ready to listen and contain it.

Durrell's Farewell from the Edge of the World

In the final paragraphs of *Pied Piper of Lovers*, Walsh Clifton offers a farewell from a secluded harbour village, or perhaps an unnamed island. He writes contentedly about life in a small cottage with his wife and children. The sun has set; he lights a lamp to complete a letter. Outside, the world is still. He describes how the waves have thrust an elbow of chalk out of its furry night-dress. He intends to walk down to the beach to bathe, and if the moon is out, he says he will be joyful.

This lyrical passage is reminiscent of the style that would define Durrell's later novels, excelling in his masterpiece *The Alexandria Quartet*. He adopts the form of the farewell letter, addressing a distant but beloved friend, as he does in *The Alexandria Quartet*. The island is both real and imagined, a geography of the mind. The peace he describes is fragile, his mood shaded by a dark, swirling melancholy from which Durrell's poetry of loss flows.

Writing, for Durrell as for many writers, emerges from *loss*. Even a grocery list is, in its way, a catalogue of what is missing. If all writing begins in *loss*, then what distinguishes a novel from a list? How profound must *the secret wound* be for the text to transcend the ephemeral and enter the domain of lasting significance?

Published in 1935, *Pied Piper of Lovers* was Durrell's debut novel, written in his early twenties. It remains his most explicitly autobiographical work. The novel traces the life of Walsh Clifton, from his birth and early years in India to his education and young adulthood in England. The novel does not offer a linear plot but rather a series of vivid episodes suffused with poetic imagery and emotional intensity.

Durrell never wrote a conventional autobiography nor maintained a diary. He told Anaïs Nin (1903–1977), who exhaustively chronicled her own life, that diary writing was a dangerous practice for him. It might, he feared, consume him entirely. What he needed to express, he insisted, could be found in his fiction and poetry. His literature, therefore, is best read as an oblique autobiography: the work of a writer who thought that direct confession would destroy the necessary distance he needed for his creativity to flourish.

Pied Piper of Lovers is composed of a prologue, three main books, and an epilogue. The narration is delivered by an undisclosed voice, seemingly omniscient yet occasionally breaking the frame to address the reader. These intrusions are subtle but significant. They evoke a spectral presence, an invisible narrator who suddenly materializes, unsettling in its very appearance. One is left to wonder: who is this voice, and where has it been all this time? These occasional disruptions hint at *the uncanny*, which Durrell's fiction frequently flirts with; something long repressed returns not in the familiar form but in an altered and eerie guise.

The prologue opens in darkness. A monsoon rages as a doctor is summoned to a remote hut where a man, John Clifton, awaits with a young woman in labour. The doctor's presence dominates the scene, with her actions portrayed in minute detail, while the mother is barely present and dies soon after childbirth. Immediately, the narrative shifts to matters of death and coffin-making. Thus, the novel begins with a triad of existential themes: birth, death, and the void in between.

The text is challenging to follow: its narrative line is elusive, its language is rich, perhaps too rich, as well as baroque and poetic. One can become lost in its sensual abundance, unsure of the story's path. This very aesthetic – lush, allusive, elliptical – would come to define Durrell's mature voice, though it would also provoke later criticism.

Interestingly, the novel is dedicated to Durrell's real-life mother, Louisa Durrell (1886–1984), yet the mother figure in the narrative dies almost immediately. As the story progresses, however, she returns, metaphorically, through the character of Brenda, John Clifton's English sister. Brenda arrives in India after the mother's death and eventually accompanies Walsh to England. She finds a home in Dulwich and offers Walsh stability in the strange new world, just as Louisa did in Durrell's life. This narrative sleight of hand, the killing of the mother only to resurrect her in the guise of the aunt, is an instance of the uncanny. The dead returns but altered. What is repressed re-emerges in disguise.

Why would Durrell make such a symbolic substitution? Why kill the mother only to bring her back to life as a childless spinster? The answer may lie in his *ambivalence* towards his parents; he blamed both, but particularly his mother, for sending him away from home too early.

Louisa Durrell was a nurturing and attentive mother. She provided the emotional foundation of Durrell's early years in India. When the time came and she had to obey his father's imperative and collaborate in the act of sending young Durrell away, even if reluctantly, it was felt as a betrayal. Not only did she terminate his years of bliss and cut him loose from the intimate connection they had, but she also agreed that he be sent away to the boarding school in Darjeeling at age 9, and then the final departure for England at 11. This marked the end of his paradise, a rupture that haunted him throughout his life.

Durrell himself later remarked that he was terribly spoilt by his mother in India. The spoiling was not mere indulgence; it was the tight bond of a child wrapped in maternal warmth. To be exiled from that warmth was shattering. He was thrust into loneliness, losing his place to his younger siblings, who remained nestled in their mother's care.

Durrell's father, concerned that his son was acquiring a lilting Indian accent, decided that he must be sent away. This was not simply a cultural gesture; it was an emotional dislocation. The paternal imperative demanded separation from the maternal, from the body and landscape of early life. Thus began the transformation of home into an ambiguous, even threatening entity.

In his final interview before his death, when he was 78 years old, not much older than Appelfeld when he wrote his autobiography, Durrell admitted that he had lived his life pretending. Even though he gave that interview in his house in the south of France, where he lived for the last 30 years of his life, he confessed to feeling he had no home or national identity. He was neither truly Indian nor truly British. Having been exiled from his homeland and mother's lap at such an early age made him, by his own admission, feel lost in the world, belonging nowhere.

The decision to send Durrell away can be read as the imposition of paternal law. This law demands that the son relinquish the mother's singular and exclusive love to become a man, a subject of the father's culture and class, an imperial version of *the Oedipal Complex*. The father sacrifices the son's sense of safety and trust in the name of a greater, imperialist legacy. It is important that he becomes a true English gentleman and not remain the free spirit he was. In doing so, the father fractures the son's identity. The Biblical story of Abraham and Isaac is an analogy of Durrell's pain of separation. Abraham is asked to give up the person he loves most, just as someone facing a deep loss or forced separation feels they are being asked to give up a part of themselves. The angel, as *a witness*, acknowledges the weight of this moment, showing that even if the sacrifice is stopped the pain and moral struggle are real and witnessed. In real life, having one's suffering acknowledged, by another person, a therapist, or even symbolically, can give meaning to the experience and help the person bear the loss. Did young Durrell have such a witness? In his case, there was no divine or earthly intervention, and the only witness was created by himself, in his literature.

In this light, the death and return of the mother in *Pied Piper of Lovers* signals more than personal loss; it is a dramatization of the emotional toll of cultural assimilation and imperial displacement. The uncanny repetition – killing and reviving the maternal – reflects Durrell's unresolved conflict, one that would echo through his adult relationships with women in his novels and real life. His later portrayals of women, at once desired and distrusted, reflect this early loss as well as his semi-conscious revenge on women, all women, following that earlier betrayal. The lost mother is both idealized and punished in fiction.

A Universe of One

From *Pied Piper of Lovers* to *The Alexandria Quartet*, Durrell constructed a world to contain the fracture at the core of his being. He created in fiction what had been lost in experience. His novels are not merely stories; they are testimonies to exile and betrayal, elegies for a vanished home. Writing became his sanctuary, the place where he was both sovereign and solitary.

In the final pages of *Pied Piper of Lovers*, Walsh declares himself a cheerful nihilist, content to believe in nothing, beholden to no one. His sensibility, he says, is the only valid laboratory. This is not indifference; it is wounded self-sufficiency. It is the declaration of someone who has lost a witness to his early life and is now trying, through literature, to recreate that gaze.

For Durrell, the act of writing was not simply expression, it was a homecoming. It was the attempt to say *I am*, even if only within the echo chamber of his own imagination.

Halfway through *Pied Piper of Lovers*, Durrell depicts the young Walsh standing on the deck of the liner that brought him to England. Gazing upon the Dover coastline, he remarks on the view to an Indian *ayah* (nanny) standing beside him. Through her eyes, the narrator conveys what may be understood as Walsh's unspoken feelings. Durrell writes that she seemed absorbed in taking in the land she had so often heard about. It is no coincidence that Durrell chose her to carry Walsh's initial impressions of the country he was meant to call home but which he would eventually learn to despise. In the figure of this beloved *ayah*, a relic from his Indian childhood paradise, the innermost textures of Walsh's emotional world are held. It is as if she, who nurtured him in the land of his birth, exists within him both as a relic but also a witness to what he has lost. Walsh turns to her and says, shyly, that he too came from the hills of Kurseong. She nods silently but does not reply. He wonders, with a tinge of bitterness, why she has shown no sign of gladness at this shared origin. He longs to speak to her of places already fading into memory, but she seems to regard him as yet another English stranger, someone with whom she shares only the coincidence of a birthplace; a land that is her home but for him merely a temporary dwelling. He bites his lip and tries to muster excitement at the sight of England. She represents that pre-verbal part of him who dwelt in that lost paradise. She remembers but cannot speak.

Why was Durrell unable to write directly about his own experience of being sent away from his home, an experience he later insisted had marked him for a life of exile and solitude? Why did he rely on a mute surrogate, the *ayah*, as a narrative vessel for this profound rupture? The answer, it seems, lies in the traumatic nature of that separation. It was an emotional wound, one that continued to haunt him and, paradoxically, fuel his creativity. The act of leaving home shaped Durrell's worldview and, in many ways, made him who he was. But perhaps it was too painful to face head-on, too formative to be rendered in literal terms.

Trauma overwhelms the individual, catching them unprepared, bypassing the symbolic order, and rendering them unable to mediate the experience through language. It collapses emotional defences and lodges itself in the depths of the individual's being, awakening archaic anxieties. Such events are particularly catastrophic when they befall infants or young children, whose ego functions and linguistic capacities are still nascent. They cannot yet deploy reason or language to defend themselves against the raw force of unmediated experience.

His adolescence in England was marked by parental absence. Having left home definitively at 11, he navigated puberty and adolescence in isolation from the daily presence of his parents. This developmental stage, crucial for identity formation and relational capacity, was therefore undertaken without the stabilizing presence of parental figures.

As discussed in Chapter Seven, adolescence involves two central developmental processes: a second phase of *separation-individuation*, the first one experienced around the age of 5, and the final resolution of the *Oedipal complex*. Both require the presence of emotionally available parents. While many adolescents manage these tasks even when physically distant from home, Durrell's particular circumstances, compounded by an earlier emotional wound, left these developmental milestones only partially negotiated.

This may explain the muted presence of the parental figures in *Pied Piper of Lovers* and the silence surrounding the pain of separation. Durrell had no witness to his early losses, no one to hear, receive, or help metabolize them. Trauma becomes catastrophic not merely due to the lack of language but due to the absence of a listening witness. Without a witness, traumatic memory remains frozen, lodged in the unconscious, reemerging through symptoms and repetition compulsions.

The absence of a detailed account of Walsh's departure – the days, weeks, and intimate gestures that composed the act of leaving – is thus not a matter of forgetfulness. It signals a lack of *containment*. There was no one to bear witness to the pain of the 11-year-old boy, and so no language could form around that rupture. Writing *Pied Piper of Lovers* as a young man, Durrell was still too close to the event and too underdeveloped in literary and psychological resources to face it directly but was able to bear testimony to its aftermath. The symbolic witness, the mature internal other, was still in the process of forming in his pursuit of literature. The past was too near; perspective had not yet fully ripened.

This absence of perspective was not only a question of developmental readiness. Durrell was denied one of adolescence's key tasks: the rebellious separation from parental figures. With his parents far away, rebellion turned inward. He became his own adversary, struggling internally against figures he could neither reject nor reconcile with. His adult life and literary themes reveal this unresolved tension, particularly in his relationships with women, marked by an oscillation between idealization and alienation. Durrell divorced three of his four wives, and his bond with his second daughter was strained. These patterns suggest an emotional immaturity rooted in an unresolved adolescence, one deprived of both external containment and internal elaboration.

Yet Durrell's creative vitality rescued him from mental dissolution. Writing became his refuge, his home, his mental laboratory. In his later novels, and already in *Pied Piper of Lovers*, one detects the slow crystallization of a worldview rooted in exile, solitude, and the sanctity of the self's interiority. His later works, most notably *The Alexandria Quartet*, offer a more nuanced and enriched exploration of these themes. But even here, in his earliest novel, the contours of his existential position are clearly drawn: a man at once joyful and despairing, detached from the world yet desperate to make sense of it through the act of writing. He aspired to a state in which he could say, *I am, and am content to be*, an ideal of ontological sufficiency unmarred by relational dependency.

In the closing pages of *Pied Piper of Lovers*, he describes himself as a *cheerful nihilist* who believes in nothing, owes nothing, and possesses no duties. His sensibility is the only meaningful domain in which true work is done. This doctrine of perfect selfishness is not mere egotism but a response to profound loss, the loss of the primary witness, the loss of the original home. Throughout his oeuvre, Durrell reworks this loss into imaginative constructions: baroque cities, psychological labyrinths, and poetic soliloquies.

In this way, Durrell's entire literary corpus can be read as a testimony to the unspeakable, an attempt to reanimate significance in the wake of early emotional rupture. His fiction creates the universe he could not inhabit as a child: a world over which he reigns with imaginative sovereignty, a world he rules beautifully, if alone. In *Pied Piper of Lovers*, as in his later work, the project is the same: to use reflection and literary invention as a way of making life intelligible. Writing became, for Durrell, not only the vehicle of self-expression but the very home to which he perpetually returned.

Freud's Experience of Leaving Home

A very different narrative concerning *leaving home* is presented by Freud. Though taking place in Europe in the same years and under similar political pressure as Appelfeld, it is a different story. It allows the reader to observe *leaving home* in a different light, finding perhaps more similarities as expressed in writing than expected.

Freud, like Durrell, did not write a comprehensive autobiography nor fiction. His writing was predominately devoted to theoretical and clinical explorations and the development of psychoanalytic theories. He was also an avid writer of letters and left behind him thousands of correspondences which testify to his mood, thoughts, and feelings in those years. He wrote to colleagues, family, and friends. It is mostly from that vast reservoir that I will narrate how Freud experienced his *leaving home*. In a sense, I posit his correspondence as his fiction.

In the introduction to this book, I use a quote from a letter Freud wrote to Princess Marie Bonaparte on 13th August, 1937, a few months before he was forced to leave his beloved Vienna, fearing the Nazis. In that quote he admits his sense of disappointment regarding the situation, leading him to sadness and depression.

Freud was already an old and not-so-well man when the Nazi party gained control in Germany and began its invasion of Austria. He was already a well-known figure in Europe, and his home at Berggasse 19 was an address many visited. His practice was well established as were his professional circles, which he kept in his endeavour to support and develop the growing psychoanalytic movement. But he was far from content.

After celebrating his 70th birthday in 1926, he confided somewhat bitterly to Marie Bonaparte that even though the Jews celebrated his person as a national hero, the university, academy, and the medical association completely ignored him. It was only the (social-democratically ruled) City of Vienna that sent him the diploma of Freedom of the City, showing the unique position he held, and he was aware of being both loved and feared in a city that felt like home yet also threatening, embodying the sense of the uncanny.

He was aware of the catastrophic political change that had gained momentum from the mid-1920s, reaching a nadir after the collapse of the financial markets and the ensuing chaos in 1929. As he wrote to the Swiss Lutheran minister Oskar Pfister (1873–1956) in May 1933 that his horizon had become darkly clouded by the events in Germany, three members of his family were already seeking ways to leave Austria.

A few months later, in 1934, after the riots in Vienna and as the situation deteriorated, he wrote to his son, Ernst Freud (1892–1970), that the future was uncertain, either Austrian fascism or the swastika. He thought that they would have to leave.

Can this moment of practical and grim awareness of the developing situation signify the beginning of leaving home for Freud? Freud was in the position of the head of the family, in charge of everybody's well-being, and thus already making provisions in his mind if the situation turned for the worse.

Still, he was able to feel somewhat safe in his home for quite a while longer. He describes his uncanny sense of being at home mixed with a feeling of the encroaching end, in a letter to the Austrian novelist Stefan Zweig (1881–1942) as late as May 1936, in which he thanked him for the speech he gave in his honour for his 80th birthday. He confessed that he felt happy in his home with his family and in particular with his daughter Anna, who satisfied his expectations as a father, and yet he couldn't reconcile himself to the wretchedness and helplessness of old age. He was looking forward with a kind of longing to the transition into nonexistence.

Freud, unlike Appelfeld and Durrell, was able to think about, remember, and recount what he was about to lose, what he would have to leave behind. As a mature individual, he was able to rely upon his supportive network of family and friends. He was able to write about his experiences while they were happening. Unlike Appelfeld and Durrell, who were only able to write about their experiences long after they took place, Freud was able to reflect on and process his daily experience and also share this with the people he chose to and receive responses.

Unlike Appelfeld and Durrell who had to store their experiences in their bodies to be recollected later through the act of writing, Freud was able to continue living his life and work almost without disturbance. But, like Appelfeld and Durrell, in those times of peril, he longed for simplicity of life.

Such thoughts helped Freud deal with the increasing difficulties. As he wrote to Stefan Zweig in October 1937, a few months before leaving Vienna, he suffered from the times they lived in and only found comfort in the feeling of solidarity with a few others who shared the values for what remained precious and incontestable. While Freud died before the horrors of the concentration camps were to fully take place, Zweig was perhaps unfortunate and sober enough to witness the disintegration of those incontestable values Freud refers to, and chose to end his own life, with his wife, on 22nd February, 1942, while living in exile in Brazil, having succeeded in leaving Europe.

As the situation worsened, Freud hinted towards the solution at hand. Referring to the historical figure of Moses, he wrote to his son Ernst in January 1938, four months before the departure to London, congratulating him on his new house in England and saying that it is typically Jewish not to renounce anything and to replace what has been lost. He thought that Moses was the first to set an example that they should learn from in those difficult times. He advised Ernst to enjoy his existence in England and stand boldly against all the misery around them. His cautious tone at that time is evident in a letter he wrote to his brother Alexander Freud (1866–1943) in Canada advising silence concerning the current situation. He was perhaps already realizing that what was to follow was indescribable.

Freud was preparing himself for leaving home, indicating that any concrete move could not come between a strong sense of belonging, being Jewish. Being Jewish accompanies him and is a link to the past and tradition, to the figure of Moses, to alleviate the sense of uprootedness inherent in the forthcoming move. When Freud wrote the letter, Marie Bonaparte was already making real efforts to secure the transit visas required for the Freud family to leave Vienna. Investing all her efforts, including vast sums of money, she was able to obtain ten visas. The act of leaving home became a reality. Her efforts began as soon as the Nazis invaded Austria in March, 1938. With Ernst Jones, in London, she arranged both his stay in England and his departure from Vienna.

Martin Freud (1889–1967), his son, wrote in his desktop diary the words *Finis Austriae* on the date of the invasion – 12th March, 1938. Despite his own awareness of this fact, Freud was reluctant at first to act upon it. It took several weeks, the temporary arrest of his daughter Anna, and the invasion of Martin's office by the Nazis to finally persuade him to accept Bonaparte's efforts. The Freud family began leaving Vienna, first Freud's daughter Mathilda and her husband and then on 3rd June Freud himself with other family members. Freud's sisters and their families stayed behind, since it was not possible to obtain visas for all of them. Freud left them sums of money, which he hoped would provide for them, but Regina Deborah Graf-Freud (1860–1943), Maria Moritz-Freud (1861–1942), Esther Adolfine Freud (1862–1943), and Pauline Regine Winternitz-Freud (1864–1942) all died in concentration camps. As Freud himself died in 1939, he did not know of their cruel fate and was spared the inevitable terrible guilt of having had to make a choice to save some of his family but not all.

During his last days in Vienna, the home he was about to leave, Freud wrote to his son Ernst in May 1938 that he was sitting inactive and helpless while Anna was running here and there coping with all the authorities, attending to all the business details. He could already imagine the journey ahead, and his only joy was in thinking about rejoining his son and dying in freedom.

Freud's home no longer felt homely and safe. It has become uncanny. He viewed his journey in Biblical terms when he wrote to Martin that he sometimes compared himself with the old Jacob, who, when a very old man, was taken by his children to Egypt. He joked that he hoped this time it wouldn't also be followed by an exodus from Egypt. Freud's reference to his Jewish background, citing Biblical figures as his role models, repeated his earlier assertion regarding the strong sense of belonging that being Jewish implies. At times when his home becomes uncanny, he returns to historical roots, showing, despite popular belief to the contrary, that he was deeply rooted within the Jewish tradition. Leaving home, leaving the concrete home of Vienna, allows Freud to return to a symbolic, primeval home, his sense of Jewish roots and belonging.

The Role of Writing as Returning Home

Clearly, this is not a comparative study. Appelfeld, Durrell, and Freud each dealt with the experience of leaving home through their writing, though under vastly different circumstances and at different stages of life. Nevertheless, I found the theme of *leaving home* and *the uncanny* common to all of them, showing just some of the myriad interpretations possible.

Appelfeld did not have a "Marie Bonaparte" to facilitate his leaving home and allow a symbolic return to historical roots. After his mother's murder, he began years of wandering. The lack of a witness, a facilitating figure, emptied Appelfeld of subjectivity. Writing became his means of processing experiences stored in his body, creating literature from the ruins of his childhood home.

Durrell's experience of being sent away for education was a total departure from his previous life. Not having gone through adolescence where he could test relationship boundaries while relying on a safe base, he remained somewhat immature, saved only by his creativity. This contributed significantly to his sense of loneliness and solitude, leading to the formation of his heraldic universe.

Freud, as a mature individual with supportive networks, was able to reflect on and process his daily experience, share it with chosen people, and receive responses. He could continue living and working almost without disturbance, but like Appelfeld, he longed for the simplicity of natural life before civilization's turmoil.

For Durrell and Appelfeld, writing served as a means of creating home where none existed or where one had been lost. Writing became the process through which they sought to form a homeland for themselves, transforming loss into creative expression.

The experience of leaving home, whether through exile, deportation, or being sent away, created in each writer a profound sense of displacement that was addressed through the act of creation. In their writing, they found not just expression but a form of return, a way of dwelling in language where physical dwelling had been denied or destroyed.

Through their literary works, Durrell and Appelfeld demonstrate that creativity often springs from the deepest wounds, that the artistic impulse emerges from the need to make meaning from loss, and that writing can serve as both testimony to suffering and the transcendence of it. Their experiences remind us that home is not merely a physical space but a psychological and emotional construct that can be rebuilt through the power of language and imagination.

Chapter 10

We Do Not Want to Be Ruled Like This

Creativity and Public Protest

In a Zoom lecture delivered in 2021, the Israeli philosopher Avi Sagi (b. 1953) argued that literature, philosophy, culture, and art are acts of saying *no* and refusing intolerable reality, thereby offering alternative possibilities. Intellectuals today must not remain silent. They must struggle to assume responsibility for the rights of everyone. Through saying *no* to oppressive measures, the possibility of being human is revealed.

This chapter addresses the ethical dilemma of how involved social workers, and other mental health professionals, can say *no* and be actively involved in the public and political arena in their society. There is a traditional claim that therapists must abstain from any public engagement in matters of the day to maintain their non-judgemental capacity, so that the client can feel free to engage in the process of *free association*. The argument is that once a client learns of the therapist's opinions, it will interfere with the process of *transference* and not allow the full containing presence they require. This was discussed to some extent in Chapter Six around the issue of *self-exposure*.

Therapists indeed need to abstain from deliberately expressing their personal political opinions to clients under almost all circumstances. Naturally, such an expression might indeed deter the client from speaking freely their own convictions. Still, to pretend that therapists do not possess political opinions or take no part in social, cultural, and political activities seems unreasonable. It would be like avoiding the very simple questions that clients often ask: *are you married? Do you have kids?* to which I recommend the therapist simply answer truthfully and plainly and then proceed to investigate the unconscious motives behind the timing of such curious questions.

In this chapter and the following one, I will describe and discuss my own social, cultural, and political involvement during times of profound social transformation. I focus on the period that began during the COVID-19 pandemic in Israel, through the current government's attempt to undermine the judicial system and the recent war in Gaza, following the murderous Hamas and its allies' attack on Israel in 2023.

Naturally, as I am focusing on current affairs that are still taking place as the final chapters of the book are written, some of the actual details included

DOI: 10.4324/9781003683162-10

may seem out of date. I hope that the essence of my argument will remain clear and relevant.

I will state at the very beginning that my motivation for actions, like my motivation for creativity, stems from a sense of *loss*. I did not choose to become socially active just because I felt like getting involved but to repair the hurt I had been experiencing. When we experience loss of any kind, as happens to all humans all the time, we have the option of dealing with it through positive actions, i.e. saying *no* to the sense of devastation and finding creative ways to regain our sense of *agency*. This of course does not suggest that we deny our loss nor the grief that follows it, but rather it gives expression to the amazing and hopeful human capacity for *recovery*.

I suggest that being a psychoanalytic social worker in Israel at present leaves us with no responsible option than to be involved. We can all chose at what stage, through what means, and how much we want to engage in such involvement. Since Israel has been and will continue to be a country under extraordinary pressures, I believe that none of its citizens have the privilege of not being actively involved. Of course, the fact that many people choose not to get involved, which is a legitimate decision, or are unable due to being too hurt, means that they are sadly relinquishing significant parts of their *agency*. This might lead to feeling powerless and frustrated, ultimately leading to symptoms of deteriorating mental health.

I will demonstrate in this chapter and in the concluding chapter that being a psychoanalytic social worker in Israel worker today extends one's capacity for action well beyond engaging in self-reflection and providing individual therapy. It can involve adopting additional paths of action that may become a vital part of the fabric of 21st-century Israeli society. This chapter will focus upon COVID-19 and the ensuing social unrest in Israel, while the next chapter will focus on the 7th October attack and the ensuing war and rise in antisemitism.

Freud and Loss: Social Symptoms of a Pandemic

The outbreak of the COVID-19 pandemic in 2020 was widely compared to an earlier global health crisis: the so-called *Spanish flu*, caused by the H1N1 influenza virus. Between 1918 and 1920, this virus swept across Europe, infecting an estimated half a billion people, approximately one-third of the world's population at the time. Like COVID-19, it progressed in successive waves, four in total, and is believed to have caused between 20 and 50 million deaths, making it far deadlier than the COVID-19 pandemic.

The term *Spanish flu* emerged not because Spain was the point of origin but because, uniquely among European nations at the time, Spain was not subject to the censorship imposed during the final stages of World War I. Spanish newspapers reported openly on the outbreak, creating the false impression that the disease originated there. In truth, the hardest-hit regions were in Central and Western Europe, including Austria, where Sigmund Freud was then living.

It was during these years that Freud composed *Beyond the Pleasure Principle*, wherein he articulated his theory of the *death drive* (Thanatos), a force he positioned alongside the *life drive* (Eros), together comprising his dual-drive model of the mind. Although later contested by proponents of Object Relations theories, this conceptual framework laid the foundation for understanding the human mind as shaped by the internalization of symbolic representations of external reality.

Within this essay, Freud famously discusses the *fort-da* game played by young children, an observation through which he inferred the emotional processes by which children manage the mother's absence. This scene would become crucial in later psychoanalytic theorizing of how *loss and absence* constitute core elements of mental life. When someone we are attached to is not physically present, whether through temporary separation or permanent loss, we revert to our internal representation of them, one with whom we maintain an ongoing bond, even if they become permanently absent through death or other reasons.

In this sense, it is not an exaggeration to suggest that the many absences we endure, beginning almost from the moment of birth, fundamentally sculpt the trajectory of our emotional development. Our inner life is what we have retained from all that has happened to us but is no longer available to us through our senses.

The child Freud observed was his grandson, Ernst Halberstadt (1914–2008), the firstborn of his beloved daughter Sophie (1893–1920), who would soon be among the many victims of the influenza pandemic. Sophie, then pregnant with her third child, fell ill in Hamburg and died on 25th January, 1920, just five days after the onset of symptoms. Her unborn child perished with her, leaving behind a grieving husband, Max, and two young sons.

Freud conveyed the devastating news to his mother, Amalia Nathansohn Freud (1835–1930), explaining that they had learned of Sophie's death through a phone call from his wife's sister. Though he initially considered travelling with his son Ernst to visit the bereaved family, he noted that his wife, Martha Bernays Freud (1861–1951), was too shattered to make the journey. And he wondered aloud: what purpose would such a visit serve, when Sophie was gone?

She was the first of his children to die. In his letter, he voiced concern for Max and the children and acknowledged the unrelenting force of grief. Mourning the loss of such a vibrant and joyful young woman, he wrote, was not only permissible but necessary. In another letter he wrote the same week to his Swiss colleague, the Reverend Oskar Pfister, Freud reflected on the helplessness he had felt as Sophie's condition worsened. Though concerned, he had not abandoned hope, for the distance made it difficult to fully grasp her situation. The family had been unable to travel to her bedside; no trains were running. Freud concluded his letter with a sombre recognition of the unmasked brutality of the times, a phrase that captures the raw anguish that shadowed both the public calamity of the pandemic and his personal grief.

The Pandemic and Social Protest in Israel

Each of these two letters, written in 1920, might just as easily have been written by someone in Israel, or nearly anywhere else in the world, in 2020. Although the viruses responsible for the Spanish flu and COVID-19 are markedly different in their biological composition, the individual, governmental, and societal responses to both pandemics reveal striking parallels. This resonance is significant: it suggests that, despite the profound sense of rupture we seemed to experience during COVID-19, the social and emotional symptoms it evoked were not entirely foreign to society. Rather, they echoed earlier patterns of response, long embedded in our collective experience, even if forgotten or unacknowledged.

Once again, society found itself grappling with a deep and disorienting disruption to the fabric of everyday life. The urgency of the moment compelled us to reflect on the ways in which we cope, both individually and collectively. Understanding our emotional and societal responses is not only a matter of historical comparison but of psychological and ethical necessity. In both pandemics, the public sphere was dramatically constricted: schools, restaurants, and cultural institutions were closed; social distancing became a normalized, even legislated, mode of behaviour, often provoking tension and resistance.

In Israel, as in many parts of the world, citizens endured multifaceted losses. The most immediate and painful was the loss of life, especially among the elderly and vulnerable. Countless others fell ill and faced long paths to recovery, both physically and emotionally.

Beyond the threat to health, the restrictions imposed by prolonged lockdowns inflicted widespread damage upon livelihoods, social cohesion, and mental well-being. The economic toll was severe, but it was matched, perhaps even surpassed, by a growing sense of social and political unrest. At moments, the psychological weight of the crisis seemed to eclipse the biological threat itself, revealing fault lines in the nation's social fabric and exposing the fragility of structures we had assumed to be stable.

In Israel those restrictions provoked public protest. In every country, the nature of the protest was essentially different. The scope of this chapter is not enough to go into what happened around the world. I focus on the Israeli popular protest movement that began in those days and is essentially still going on, more than five years later.

I found myself drawn into active participation, first just attending protests, then becoming more actively involved in organizing them, as well as documenting them with my camera and sharing my pictures and videos on social media. The deeper my involvement, the more concerned I became with the question as to whether I was crossing professional boundaries by exposing my political convictions in a way that might feel intrusive to my clients and students. I am still concerned and believe that being aware of the possible infringements allows me to deal with them in a responsible and ethical way. In a sense, I have crossed again the same line which I have crossed in the past by publishing prose and poetry since 2000. I was prepared to acknowledge possible reactions to this on-going personal exposure through *transference* in the therapy room, as I have demonstrated throughout this book.

The issues that brought many Israelis to protest have shifted over time, but the underlying concern remains the same: a deep mistrust of how the elected right-wing, conservative government manages Israel's affairs, both at home and abroad. There was one year after an election when a liberal government took office in 2021, but it didn't last long. Today, Israel is once again governed by a right-wing conservative government, which has been the norm for most of the past 34 years.

The protest I am referring to as an example has been taking place across the streets of Israel, with a particular focus on Balfour Street in Jerusalem, the official residence of the Israeli prime minister. Tens of thousands of individuals have participated, representing diverse groups, some of which emerged spontaneously, such as the *Black Flags Protest, Crime Minister*, and others. Beyond that, every Friday evening and Saturday night, demonstrations take place at hundreds of intersections throughout the country, as well as in front of the prime minister's private residence. More recently, since the war in Gaza evolved into what some view as an unjustified war whose sole purpose is to maintain the current government in power, these protests have become less consensual. But still, they persist.

These are not conventional protest events. True, they include familiar elements of public demonstrations in Israel: stages with speakers, organized marches, rhythmic chants, and, inevitably, a strong police presence, at times veering into excessive force and raising suspicions of politically motivated behaviour. What, in my view, distinguishes these protests from previous political demonstrations in Israel, including the 2011 social protest movement, is the distinctly carnivalesque atmosphere. Anyone who has visited one of the protest hubs, particularly Balfour, could not fail to be struck by the presence of clowns, street performances, large puppets, music, and even meditation circles. Even members of Netanyahu's family, unable to ignore this dimension, mockingly referred to the demonstrators as *aliens*, referencing their circus-like attire and theatrical displays.

But what is the aim of this protest movement, beyond the repeated calls at these gatherings for the resignation of Benjamin Netanyahu, who has been the democratically elected prime minister, with some gaps, since 1995 and is currently standing trial for charges of bribery, fraud, and breach of trust? Ostensibly, the answer to this question is self-evident to any informed citizen in Israel. It dominates headlines and news broadcasts daily. However, I wish to offer a slightly different interpretation of this mass mobilization and its underlying objectives.

Precisely the carnivalesque element of the protest, its theatricality, creativity, and the participation of thousands from across the sociopolitical spectrum of Israeli society, suggests that the movement is responding not only to the visible economic and political crises. Rather, it points to a deeper, structural rupture within Israeli society. The symbolic presence of *a carnival* at the heart of a popular uprising reveals that the multitudes participating, alongside hundreds of thousands more who have supported the movement from a distance, whether due to COVID-19 in 2020–2021 and now due to the on-going war, are animated by a shared, if largely unconscious, desire for profound systemic change.

We Do Not Want to Be Ruled This Way

It is perhaps a cliche to say that those who fail to learn from the past are doomed to repeat it. Still, cliches hold within them a sense of truth, though one which has been repeated too often and not always in the right context. I trust that this cliche resonates with Freud's concept of the *repetition compulsion*, whereby repressed conflicts or unresolved traumatic material persistently seek expression, through symptoms, slips of the tongue, dreams, and the recursive patterns of everyday life. What remains unintegrated does not disappear; instead, it returns, often disguised, insisting upon recognition.

To attempt a more distant perspective on what is going on currently, I turn a diachronic eye towards Albert Camus's 1947 novel *The Plague*, which offers profound insight into the psychological and social reverberations of a mass epidemic as representing social disease, which in turn brings out the multitudes onto the street calling for change.

While the novel is loosely based on the 1849 cholera outbreak in Oran, Algeria, Camus transposes the narrative to a fictional outbreak in the same city during the 1940s. In one of its most haunting passages, he writes of the townspeople, who, amid mounting despair, struggle to retain a sense of inner freedom. He recounts how some even manage to imagine they are still acting as free men because they think they can still choose. Yet, by mid-August, he writes, chaos is in charge. There are no longer individual choices, only a collective ordeal. The plague, which all fear, creates an ever-growing sense of estrangement and alienation.

Thematic currents of freedom, fate, individual agency, and the tension between the self and society, central to Camus's entire philosophical oeuvre, are vividly present throughout *The Plague*. Written during World War II, the novel bears unmistakable allegorical resonances with the Nazi occupation of Europe. It marks a turning point in Camus's intellectual trajectory: having previously advanced an absurdist outlook in *The Myth of Sisyphus*, he moves towards a more politically committed position, one that calls for active resistance to oppressive forces.

For Camus, the confrontation with an existential threat does not negate meaning; rather, it opens a space in which human beings may choose to endow their lives with significance. Meaning is not discovered; it is created through struggle. Without such resistance, the individual risks becoming a passive object, swept along by impersonal forces. In contrast, through action, solidarity, and moral engagement, one may reclaim a sense of autonomy.

This existential ethic bears direct relevance to the practice of social work. The imperative to not give in to despair and encourage empowerment lies at the heart of social work, certainly as I have been practising and teaching it: when we face individuals and communities in states of marginalization or despair, our task is not only to bear witness to suffering but also to cultivate hope and agency. Like Camus's plague victims, our clients may find themselves facing forces beyond their control. Yet within this confrontation lies the possibility, however fragile, of renewed dignity, meaning, choice, and regaining s sense of *agency.*

In my opinion, at the heart of public struggle for change, regardless of political affiliation, lies Michel Foucault's (1926–1984) statement: *We do not want to be ruled like this.* This declaration, which appears in his 1997 essay *What Is Critique?* encapsulates a basic drive behind all social protest, an impulse to which social workers, mental health workers, and citizens must remain deeply attuned.

Foucault's statement rests on two interdependent principles. The first is the very existence of governance as a system designed to structure the relationship between the sovereign and the people. The second concerns the way this governance is exercised under particular historical and social conditions. The outcry w*e do not want to be ruled like this* emerges from a sense of existential threat to democratic life. This threat is neither new nor temporary; rather, it is rooted in the deep historical processes that have shaped modern society.

This chapter cannot fully capture the complexity of Israel's situation, but some points can be made. Jewish immigration to Israel was driven both by the urgent need to find a safe political place for the Jews scattered all over the world and haunted by antisemitism, especially after Holocaust, and by the long-held belief that Israel was the natural homeland for Jews after centuries of exile. What makes this return complicated is that the land was already inhabited by another ethnic group, the Palestinians, and surrounded by hostile Arab countries. Managing such a complex political and geographic reality has shaped Israel's forms of government and often caused public unrest. Israel is still working to define both its internal ethnic boundaries and its external borders. Living with ongoing internal tensions and real external threats has led to challenging and sometimes unstable governance.

The fact that governments exist during times of crisis shows how closely organization, knowledge, and power are connected, and how they are put into practice. As Foucault points out, power always generates resistance; there can be no control without pushback, and counter-movements are inevitable. From this perspective, the mass protests during the COVID-19 pandemic, and now during the war Israel has been engaged in in Gaza, Lebanon, Syria, Iran, and Yemen during the last couple of years, were in fact an integral part of the system they were rising against; they were part of the very structures they challenged. Protest and governance are not opposites, they influence each other. In other words, a government may not exist without some form of resistance.

The second point is about the way we are governed. This idea comes from Foucault's studies of 18th-century European political systems, especially in France and Germany, where religion played a major role. Early forms of pastoral power and disciplinary governance became models for modern democratic governments. In Israel, where religion and state are deeply intertwined, these historical roots are especially relevant and complex.

Foucault also has a unique way of thinking about history. He sees time as uneven: things change, but the past never completely disappears. Once there was a king; now there is a republic. But the king could, in some sense, return. This folding of time is where history is born, where people become subjects, and where governance works not only through laws and commands but also by shaping how people think and regulate themselves.

In *The Order of Things*, Foucault describes a major shift in human knowledge at the end of the 18th century. What had seemed like a continuous cultural order suddenly broke into new ways of understanding the world. This kind of disruption continues today, reflected in the extreme fragmentation of Israeli politics, where consensus is replaced by division and confusion.

Could it be, then, that part of the deep unease felt by many Israeli citizens, especially in the face of rising charismatic, anti-democratic leaders, stems from an incomplete historical transition? Might the symbolic movement from monarchy to democracy never have been fully realized in Israel, leaving a residual emotional yearning for a omnipotent leader, a king, who would promise unity in the face of disorder? Has Benjamin Netanyahu's rule, and the opposition it provokes, fitted right into that constellation?

Foucault describes a major shift in how people understand the world, which happened as society moved from the classical, monarchical age to the modern, democratic age. He looks at this change in three areas: work and the economy, science, and language.

In the economy, work used to be understood mainly by the things it produced, goods or products. In the modern view, work itself, time, effort, and human energy, becomes the main focus of analysis. It's no longer just about what is made but about the process of labour itself and its connection to production.

In science, classification also changes. Earlier systems focused on what things looked like on the outside. Modern science instead looks at internal structures and the dynamic forces inside them, such as energy and resistance. Foucault sees this as similar to his idea of power: forces never exist alone but always in relation to other forces.

In language, the shift is equally profound. Classical linguistics focused on words as direct labels for objects. Modern linguistics, however, studies how words relate to each other, through syntax, inflection, and differences within the system. Meaning comes from these relationships, not from direct naming. This change brings history and social context into language and thought. Protest slogans, graffiti, and chants are examples: they don't just express anger; they challenge existing meanings and create new possibilities. Each act of protest becomes a way of rewriting the social order.

From all this, Foucault asks a bigger question: what makes an event important enough to study, rather than just a random occurrence? For him, an event is a break in normal understanding, when appearances no longer match reality. It's a moment that reveals hidden forces, emotions, and conflicts. The clear, confident way of knowing from the classical age collapses, replaced by a view of the world and the self as complex, conflicted, and constantly changing.

Based upon such complex theorizing, the public protest in Israel over the last few years is far deeper than a mere opposition to the current government. Its deeper stratum reflects an elemental conflict between a democratic ethos, committed to upholding constitutional principles such as the separation of powers, and an emergent monarchical impulse, one that supports the concentration of unchecked authority in a charismatic and populist figure who has decide to abuse the democratic process that has allowed them to rule.

These grassroots movements have revealed themselves not merely as political protests in the conventional sense but as a profound challenge to the very structure of governance. The central question has shifted: it is no longer simply who will win the next election but whether democratic elections will retain meaning at all, or whether we are witnessing the rise of a new regime, one sustained by intricate alliances of capital, ideology, and authority, divorced from institutional accountability.

The cry of *we are not going to be ruled like this*, no longer refers to a shared critique within a commonly accepted regime. Instead, it articulates a widening rift, between liberal rationality and a traditionalist approach based upon rigid and conservative values. This tension is made visible, even palpable, in the carnivalesque dimension of modern protest: a theatre of dissent that disrupts conventional forms and reframes resistance through satire, and play.

This is not merely a semantic, epistemic, or power-based crisis. It addresses the call for a formation of new relationships between individuals and society, after the cries of alienation, disillusionment, and longing for reconnection. Foucault offers no prescriptive answers, only a diagnosis of the alienation that arises when individuals and communities become estranged from the structures that once gained their trust. This alienation remains profoundly present in Israeli society today, and social workers, uniquely situated at the nexus of public systems and private lives, are in a vital position to engage with and challenge it.

The fissures in the fabric of Israeli society that are being exposed through the popular protest were not creates by the outbreak of COVID-19. They were there to begin with, perhaps as an inevitable part of establishing a new state which is composed of very diverse Jewish immigration from dozens of different countries into a land that was already the home of indigenous Muslim, Christian and Druze communities.

The pandemic did confront all citizens regardless of their ethnic affiliation with the fact that what was once familiar had become tinged with existential threat. Everybody's personal and collective coping strategies for the daily goings-on in Israel – ranging from adaptation to resistance, which testified to a remarkable human capacity to survive – were once again challenged at precisely the moment when solidarity and cooperation were most needed to confront public health and economic emergencies. Long-standing fractures within Israeli society – ethnic, religious, class-based, and ideological – reemerged with renewed force. The pandemic did not create these fissures; it amplified them, exposing them as open wounds in the national body. What surfaced was not only protest against specific policies but a social symptom, a rupture in the symbolic order demanding redress.

The mass mobilization of people into the streets, their reclamation of public space, their refusal to remain passive spectators to political corruption, signifies an insistence on political subjectivity. When citizens step out of their homes, join strangers, and march with a shared voice, they are engaging in more than opposition; they are redefining citizenship, making themselves visible in a political world that often renders them invisible.

The Carnival

Popular protests exhibit similar and familiar rituals: speeches, chants, marches, boards with slogans. A police presence, often escalating into confrontation and, at times, violence, has become an expected part of the routine. One element stands out and is frequently misunderstood or dismissed: *the carnival*. At nearly every protest, alongside the slogans and megaphones, appear clowns, jugglers, street performers, giant puppets, and meditation circles. To an unsympathetic onlooker, particularly one ideologically opposed, these elements may seem naïve, unserious, even delusional.

Yet it is precisely this carnival presence that reveals the most subversive core of the protest. Far from being incidental or merely decorative, the *carnival* embodies the emotional, symbolic, and unconscious dimensions of political dissent. It brings together people from across the social and political spectrum, dissolving rigid categories and enacting what Bakhtin called the temporary liberation from the prevailing truth. The carnival mocks authority while pointing towards a new order. It collapses binaries, serious and silly, real and imagined, ruler and ruled, into a space of radical potential.

The traditional role of *the jester*, perhaps the main protagonist in *the carnival*, is to hold a mirror to power, to say what cannot otherwise be said. So too does the carnival serve as a mirror, reflecting not only the absurdities of the existing regime but also the desire for transformation. Through music, costumes, laughter, and satire, protestors say: what once felt familiar now feels alien. What once felt safe is now threatening. *We no longer accept being rules like this.*

Such a call contains a profound yearning, not only for a different kind of government but for a different kind of relation to the world, one in which meaning is co-created, power is answerable, and subjectivity is not colonized by ideology or despair. Social workers, attuned to these hidden dimensions of human suffering and resilience, are called not only to observe these movements but to stand with them, to bear witness, to amplify, and, where possible, to transform.

Bakhtin recognized the subversive and unifying power of civic protest in *the carnival*. He argued that the heart of the carnival lies in its transgression of established social boundaries and the creation of a radically new order of interpreting familiar social signs. Within the carnival, what is ordinarily marginal is rendered central; that which is forbidden, such as overt expressions of love and intimacy, is not only permitted but celebrated. Marginalized and disenfranchised groups ascend to prominence, while rulers and authorities become objects of ridicule.

For Bakhtin, the carnival is indispensable to the social fabric, offering a wild, anarchic, and liberatory alternative to the regimented routines defined by hierarchy and alienation. The marginalized individual is freed from both imagined and real chains and claims a central position. Traditional instruments of power, such as the police, are subjected to mockery, parody, and contempt. The vibrant spectacles and creative symbols that flood public squares act to dissolve everyday social barriers; differences of sex, race, and age temporarily dissolve, yielding space for a new social being grounded in free contact and liberation.

The carnival's essence is not merely to overturn reality; more profoundly, it seeks to reconcile what appears to be contradictory, forging a new social reality where alienation between the individual and their surroundings is dissolved.

From this vantage point, the path to a renewed social contract appears to become more possible, attentive to our shared existential anxieties. Just as an individual's resilience is tested amid crisis, so too is the society we inhabit. In moments of threat, the fissures and developmental cracks within the individual mind become exposed. When left unaddressed, these fractures manifest in pathological responses, both inward and outward. Israeli society as a collective mind, composed of myriad individuals and groups, reveals during crises the accumulated fissures.

Only time will tell whether the current upheavals will strengthen values of liberty, equality, and fraternity underpinning Israel and other modern democratic societies, or whether it will precipitate pathological social conditions characterized by fear, restriction, and hatred.

Nothing ever truly disappears or ends; rather, it sinks into forgotten depths, awaiting a chance to return, leaving *traces* behind. Even when we believe we have vanquished the plague or overcome our enemies, victory is never absolute. The next cycle is always possible. We know this concerning individual psychotherapy, and it is obviously true for societies at large. Freud named it *the compulsion to repeat*.

Viktor Frankl, a student of Freud and founder of logotherapy, wrote in *Man's Search for Meaning*, written after surviving the Holocaust, that mental health depends on an ongoing tension between what one has already achieved and what one must still strive for, between what one is and what one can be. Conflict, he argued, is essential to mental health; the illusion of a final, tensionless balance or homeostasis is both futile and harmful. Rather, the striving towards meaningful goals is what sustains mental health, not the childish fantasy of discharging all tension at any cost.

To conclude, what can we do? Hannah Arendt, herself a refugee of Nazi persecution, in her monumental *The Human Condition* distinguishes three categories of human activity in the modern era: *labour*, defined as all acts aimed at immediate survival; *work*, as the creation of durable objects and tools to serve survival; and *action*, the sphere of human relations and political engagement.

It is my hope, indeed, my conviction, that it is *action*, in Arendt's sense, that grants us meaning in a world saturated with uncertainty, even if its outcomes are transient. Participating actively in public life outside the therapy room, in whatever form each person chooses, enables us to practise our independence and freedom. Some will take to the streets in protest; others will turn inward, towards family and home. Some may seek spiritual work while others embrace political and social activism. Everyone must answer the call of their own heart. Above all, the imperative is clear: not to remain silent in the face of uncertainty and dread but to rise and participate in the effort of shaping our collective future.

Creative Social Work

One of the strengths of social work practice nowadays is the use of creative means in individual therapy. In the past, creative means such as use of the visual arts, drama, movement, photography, and other forms were usually confined to rehabilitation and community work. In recent decades in Israel, more mental health practitioners and social workers are using such methods to supplement verbal methods with a wider range of clients and contexts.

Being a creative social worker does not mean becoming an art therapist. These are two different disciplines that might share many ideas and practices but are distinctly different. Creative social workers are psychotherapists who have personal access to and use of a variety of intervention techniques that stretch beyond the verbal ones as suggested by psychoanalytic psychotherapy.

Social workers who use creative interventions during psychotherapy do this without compromising the basic tenets of psychoanalytic psychotherapy. I have been leaning towards this expansion, this disruption, for many years. Part of the process that I went through during these years of protest was allowing myself to give fuller legitimacy to more creative forms of intervention in the face of traditional methods, which are still relevant but need to be reconsidered. This was a part of my response to the call: *we do not want to be ruled like this.*

After years of incorporating these methods into university courses and clinical practice, like other social workers in Israel, such as Ephrat Huss at Ben-Gurion University, I was able to contribute to the launch of a master's programme in clinical social work with a specialization in the arts at the University of Haifa in 2024, where these ideas are both taught and applied in practice.

Chapter 11

Beyond Professional Boundaries

Antisemitism and 7th October, 2023

The profession of social work inherently involves active engagement with the social environment in which one lives and carries a deep ethical imperative: to be fully active in society in order to promote and uphold the professional and personal values one holds dear.

Being ethically concerned about my involvement in what I do as an adult began when I did my compulsory miliary service in the IDF in the early 1980s, when I witnessed some events which have left an everlasting toxic impression upon me, and I refused to take part in what I believed was wrong. Later when I was writing my final essay for my BA (Honours) degree in Photography at Trent Polytechnic in Nottingham, England in the mid-1980s, well before I even thought of training as a social worker and psychotherapist, I chose to study the works of four photographers who took pictures before and during World War II. The photographers' treatment of what they witness often tends to be couched in an aura of being realistic and truthful, which is used to protect them from scrutiny and from suspicion of bias. The resulting authority of the photographer blurs the important distinction between what the event is and what its representation is and obscures the role that the photographer/observer plays in both.

I was preoccupied with what these photographers knew and how much impact their sometimes horrific photographs had. Studying the works of Margaret Bourke-White (1904–1971) and George Rodger (1908–1995), both photojournalists, and Joe Heydecker (1916–1997), a German officer, and Roman Vishniac (1897–1990), a Jewish photographer, taught me a great deal about photography, the search for truth, and keeping testimony and guilt. It also taught me a great deal about being *a concerned citizen*, which is perhaps the real title for this concluding chapter.

Ever since, in Israel and in the UK, I have found myself active in various social arenas, trying to make a difference while at the same time being fully aware of my relative impact. I am still guided by the proverb in the Jewish Pirkei Avot tractate (the ethics of the Fathers) which says that *you are not obliged to complete your mission, but you are not permitted to stop trying while being alive.*

DOI: 10.4324/9781003683162-11

7th October, 2023

Like all other Israelis, I awoke on Saturday 7th October, 2023 to what would turn out to be the worst living nightmare of my lifetime to date.

From 6:30 am, a barrage of at least 4,300 rockets was launched into Israel's southern border by Hamas. Approximately 6,000 Gazans breached the border at 119 locations, attacking military bases and massacring 1,195 civilians and soldiers in 21 communities and army installations. Inhumane acts of barbarity were committed, including sexual atrocities.

On that day, 251 Israelis, including children, old people, and women, were kidnapped and taken to Gaza.

Israel retaliated and counter-attacked Gaza. Many thousands of Palestinians were killed, and Gaza has been left in ruins. Since that morning, Israel has also been attacked by missiles from Lebanon, Yemen, and Iran. It successfully defended itself but incurred severe damage and many casualties. At the time of this book going to print, a ceasefire was agreed upon with the intervention of the American president, Donald Trump (b. 1946), raising some hope that perhaps a more stable settlement towards permanent peace might be reached.

After the Holocaust, when six million Jews were murdered by the Nazis and their allies, the establishment of the Jewish state of Israel in 1948 was founded on the belief that *it would never happen again*. Jews will never again be massacred like helpless animals. I, having researched and written about my family's roots in Europe, a family decimated by the Holocaust, was certain that I would never feel the helplessness I imagined in horror my dead relatives felt when they were rounded up from their home in Thessaloniki and Paris and massacred in Auschwitz.

Well, it seems we were wrong. The images of what Hamas terrorists were doing during those hours before the Israeli army responded was as bad. Not only were they committing atrocious and sexual war crimes against innocent men, women, and children, they proudly shared *live feeds* of their barbaric acts on social media.

They were taking pride in the war crimes they were committing with the purpose of causing deep fear and trauma, as part of their blatantly expressed directive to eradicate Israel.

The scope of this book, or its purpose, is not sufficient to analyse in more detail the events of the war, which is still raging as I am writing these lines, but suffice to say that the notion of human evil again surfaced in Israel and the world and comparisons to what the Nazis did were inevitable. It took 843 days from the Hamas attack until all hostages, living and deceased, were returned. Hostages were kept in inhuman conditions, and Hamas was releasing photos and videos showing them to be malnourished and begging for help, as part of their propaganda. Throughout the time they were held by Hamas, no Red Cross visits were permitted by Hamas.

The state of the displaced civilian population in Gaza is unbearable. Many thousands suffered hunger. Many buildings, including historic sites and hospitals, were demolished. The horrendous conditions in Gaza are attributed to intentional Israeli military pressure, the breakdown of distribution systems, Hamas' continuous exploitation of their own people, and the continuation of the war beyond any reason apart from the political survival of the leadership on both sides. To date, thousands of Palestinians are still buried underneath the ruins of buildings destroyed by IDF attacks, preventing their families from burying them and properly mourning their loss. In some ways, it seems at this point as if the war is being conducted between two criminal organizations who pay no heed to the suffering of the population they are submitting to their reign of terror.

Meanwhile, international calls for the establishment of an in dependent Palestinian state are also growing. Without denying the severe stress and damage caused to innocent people in Gaza, it seems that the world has shifted its focus and is ignoring the atrocities and lethal intentions of Hamas and its allies to eliminate Israel and is now targeting Israel as the sole perpetrator of injustice. Again, Jessica Benjamin's *mutual recognition* imperative is invaluable here but at the moment seems to be often ignored by the avid and fanatic drive for destruction and revenge. The human suffering around me at the time of writing this chapter is unrelenting.

Regression to revenge has become quite a common defence mechanism amongst many Israelis. Anything else is considered *defeatism*. I argue that defeatism is the inability to admit loss. Out of shame, anger, and fear, we refuse to accept defeat as an option. The fear is that once we admit to losing, recovery will be impossible. After the massacre of 7th October, instead of pausing to mourn or absorb what happened, the loss was quickly transformed into the fuel for a future victory. Defeat was declared unacceptable, so anger and shame were redirected into determination. But in doing so, grief was bypassed. The pain, the humiliation, the helplessness were pushed aside, treated as obstacles rather than truths that need to be faced.

The problem is that emotions do not disappear when ignored. They shape actions whether we acknowledge them or not. When we use them only as fuel for battle, we risk becoming like ghosts, half alive, stuck in a corridor that never leads to a real reckoning. War then becomes a way of delaying facing mourning and loss. Yet sooner or later, that reckoning must come. Facing the emotional dimensions of loss is not weakness; it is necessary for healing. Otherwise, we remain suspended in endless struggle, fighting outward battles to avoid the inner ones.

Despair is Not an Option

Immediately after the attack of 7th October, I knew I had to face my mourning and regain my sense of *agency* and not regress into toxic areas of seeking revenge. As I was too old to rejoin the army in my capacity as a mental health officer, which was my last position while I was doing my reserve military service, I turned my energies to other channels where I had already been active.

As a therapist, I offered pro-bono focused dynamic therapy to about ten families of survivors and evacuees. Such work enabled me to find and offer hope to people whose lives were scarred on that morning. I heard very harrowing stories of the ways people survived and testimonies about those who did not survive. I felt privileged in a sense in my capacity as a witness to those tales, helping others to regain their familiar defence strategies and begin thinking about recovery and rehabilitation.

There were thousands of mental health experts like me around the country, setting up provisional therapy areas near the borders and in the evacuation centres and offering voluntary support to the many thousands of families, including young children. It took a while for the official state agencies to kick into action, and now such practices are running more smoothly, proving daily care for the many survivors, bereaved, and relatives of the hostages and the wounded, body and soul.

The second area I involved myself in so that my sense of concern could recover from the shock was video testimonies. I joined an ad hoc voluntary group of cinematographers, archivists, and social activists, who set out to document on film the testimonies of the survivors, *Edut 710* (Testimony 710). As I had some expertise in video editing, I edited about 150 such testimonies during a period of ten months beginning in January 2024. Again, I felt privileged in being able to utilize my skills for such an important enterprise, which was beginning to model itself on what Yad Vashem did with testimonies of Holocaust survivors. It also reflected my work on my own family's history of Holocaust survival, work which I have written about extensively in the past.

The third area of voluntary work was in joining a national network of volunteers, *Haogen (Abchor)*, that support the families of the soldiers who were called up to service. I, with some of my colleagues, managed to assemble a group of more than 100 volunteers, who help with domestic chores like cooking, shopping, and childcare for more than 200 families in my town. We were able to relieve some of the burden of these families. This work is still going on.

Lastly, the fourth area of voluntary activity is my involvement in the *Road to Recovery*, already mentioned in Chapter Eight. The *Road to Recovery* voluntary organization was founded by a friend of mine whose brother was murdered by Hamas terrorists in 1995, soon after the Oslo Accords were signed. Instead of seeking revenge, he joined an Israeli Palestinian group of bereaved individuals aiming to hold a mutual space for grieving and for working towards a better future where all ethnic groups can live together in Israel. He then founded R2R, the sole aim of which is to take sick Palestinian children and adults to lifesaving medical treatment in Israeli hospitals. Since then, everyday hundreds of Jewish volunteers drive these Palestinians from the checkpoints in the West Bank and the Gaza Strip to hospitals to receive such care. Despite a short break immediately after 7th October, these activities have continued in full steam. For me, this signifies the way forward. Finding ways of forming dialogues and daily meetings between the Jewish and Palestinian populations as a marker towards a better future.

I was writing this chapter soon after returning from a conference of the World Congress of Psychotherapy (WCP) in Vienna, where I gave a lecture concerning such issues. I am a board member of WCP and represent the Israeli Association of Psychoanalytic Psychotherapy (IAPP). During the conference, I had many meaningful conversations with other delegates, including Iranians, Lebanese, Saudis, and Moroccans, where it was shown, again, that it does not take much to form trusting and operational contacts with people with whom you may not agree on everything. It was another very important sign that my concern for peace bears fruit and that I have regained my sense of agency in the world and not only as an individual psychotherapist.

Has Antisemitism Ever Disappeared?

Almost immediately after the 7th October massacre, in some kind of a *reaction formation*, there has been a dramatic rise in virulent antisemitism around the world. In Ireland, for instance, already on 8th October there was a Pro-Palestine rally without giving equal voice against the atrocities committed the previous day by Hamas. I shall not go into whether the *Pro-Palestine* demonstrations are an expression of antisemitism or legitimate protest against the policies of the current Israeli government. Nor will I explore why it is that so many Western groups rally for Palestinian rights but ignore the oppression of so many other minorities throughout the world. This is not what this book is about. I do make the claim that despite the fact that Israel does have to answer for its part in the continuation of the conflict, there is an underlying suspicious that the attacks in the West on Israeli policies and tactics are also fuelled by well disguised antisemitic sentiments.

Since the Hamas attack on Israel on 7th October, 2023, there has been a marked global surge in antisemitic incidents. These events have included harassment, vandalism, and physical violence targeting Jewish individuals and institutions, often under the guise of anti-Israel sentiments. The spike in antisemitism has been documented across various regions, including North America, Europe, and the Middle East.

In the US there was a 337% rise in reported antisemitic incidents between 7th October and 7th December, 2023, compared to the same period in 2022. Synagogues, Jewish-owned businesses, and Holocaust memorials have been defaced or attacked. Examples include Molotov cocktail attacks on synagogues in Germany, vandalism of Jewish cemeteries in Nicaragua, and physical violence against individuals displaying Israeli symbols. In addition, antisemitic rhetoric has surged on social media, with posts often blending Holocaust denial, conspiracies, and extreme anti-Zionism. Some messages explicitly call for violence against Jews. Universities in the US and Europe have witnessed a sharp increase in antisemitic incidents, with many Jewish students reporting feelings of insecurity and pressure to conceal their identities. In countries like South Africa, Spain, and Canada, protests against Israel have frequently featured explicitly antisemitic rhetoric, equating Jews with Nazis or glorifying historical persecution.

As I will make clear in my analysis, my position adopts what Jessica Benjamin advocates in her 2018 book *Beyond Doer and Done To*.

Jessica Benjamin explains that when two people see their relationship only as a fight between *a doer* (the one in control) and the *done-to* (the one who suffers control), they get stuck in a cycle of domination and resistance. Each side feels like it must either win or lose. This way of relating is destructive because it leaves no space for *mutual recognition*, seeing the other as a real, separate human being with needs, fears, and hopes.

The Israeli–Palestinian conflict often plays out in this *doer/done-to* dynamic. Each side experiences itself as the one being harmed, controlled, or threatened while viewing the other as the aggressor. This fuels endless cycles of violence, retaliation, and mistrust.

Benjamin's idea suggests that the only way out is for both peoples to move beyond this rigid frame and towards mutual recognition. That means recognizing the other not just as an enemy but as a community with its own history, suffering, and desire for safety and dignity. Mutual recognition does not erase conflict, but it opens the door for negotiation, coexistence, and repair. Instead of being locked into *winner versus loser*, both people could begin to imagine a future in which they live side by side as subjects, not as enemies.

The origins of antisemitism are too beyond the scope of this chapter. I will, however, begin my study by scrutinizing modern antisemitism in Freud's lifetime, as he is such a pivotal figure in my study. In 1873 Freud began his medical studies in Vienna. In May that year, the Austrian stock market crashed, causing mass bankruptcies and bank failures. The antisemitic reactions in the press blamed Jewish conspiracy as the cause for the crisis. This is cited by Peter Gay (1923–2015), Freud's biographer, as one of the key moments of his Jewish self-awareness.

One could say then that Jewish self-awareness would not exist without antisemitism. However, realizing that one's sense of identity, or at least a component of it, can be the cause of such hatred from one's environment can be quite a severe blow to one's sense of security in the world.

Freud experienced antisemitism throughout his life. In several of his letters, he referred to antisemitic people as rabble. He wrote in *The Future of an Illusion* in 1927 that every civilization is erected upon coercion and renunciation of instinct and therefore implies that there are destructive, anti-social and anti-cultural parts in everyone. Antisemitism, then, from a Freudian point of view, is an inborn, primitive, and destructive instinct that can be held back and suppressed only through societal measures. As such, it is no different from other destructive instincts that are directed towards whatever, or whomever, it is that stands in the way of satisfying the drive to pleasure, such as misogyny or other forms of racism.

Destructive instincts are not judged from a moral point of view in the Freudian theory. They are part of human nature and have their origins and partial survival justifications from previous human eras such as the hunter-gatherer culture or other periods where seemingly only force could be used to protect one's abode and family from hostile natural and human forces. The Freudian assumption that human life is motivated both by innate libidinal and destructive forces outlines developmental junctions where the clash between the two drives must be elevated and be reasoned with if one wishes to conduct *a civilized and rational life* and obey a humanly enforced order, as has been the goal of liberal and democratic societies over the last few centuries.

Going a bit deeper and into the intrapsychic dimension, I suggest that it is possible to examine antisemitism in the light of the Freudian notion of the *Oedipus complex*. Failing in the Oedipal challenge, which means *not* relinquishing the narcissistic notion that one is the centre of the world, leaves the individual, or a certain community, craving for the return of the idyllic connection with the primary caretaker. Such an individual is forever locked in an endless pursuit of trying to recreate the conditions for such a focus. Naturally, this cannot be achieved and leaves the individual with unresolved aggression towards whom they think deprived them of that perfect love. One is then caught in a cycle of seeking objects towards whom they can project this aggression and revenge for their loss – revenge taken on a future partner, their children, a part of themselves and most easily on other individuals or groups that seem to be behaving in ways that are annoying and different to one's own.

The Jews, as individuals and as a racial and ethnic group, offer perfect targets and candidates for such a *projection*. Always alien and until 1948 without a political home they could call their own, always bearing and practising a different religion and culture, they can be easily blamed for all that is wrong in one's life. Rather than take responsibility for one's own natural failings, it is better to blame the Jews.

A disclaimer: other minorities too are of course subjected to the same process of projection. The Jews as such are not unique in this sense nor suffer more than other minorities. I focus upon the Jewish fate without claiming that other minorities suffer less.

The Jews and Jewish way of life, with their insistence of maintaining their separateness and uniqueness, was always a challenge to the communities where they lived. Jews refused to assimilate willingly (often they were coerced) and abandon their way of life, including but not only their religious ceremonies. The position they therefore carved, or sought to uphold, for themselves in the host communities was complex: on the one hand a wish or demand to be treated as equals, and on the other a demand to be allowed to lead their own ways of life, which often stood in contrast to their neighbours.

This was of course most prominent from a religious aspect, where Jews living in Christian countries were blamed for the crucifixion of Jesus Christ. It is generally believed that Jews lived under Islamic rule as *dhimmis* (protected but subordinate non-Muslims). While they faced discrimination and had to pay the *jizya* tax, their status was often better than under Christian rule in Europe.

Guilt and Ambivalence

I now come to a thorny junction. If what Jessica Benjamin writes is true, can the Jews be blamed, at least in part, for the hatred directed against them? To rephrase the question, are Jews themselves expressing antisemitic criticism against Israel?

Jessica Benjamin's idea in *Beyond Doer and Done To* is that human relationships often get trapped in a cycle where one side is the *doer* and the other is the *done-to*. Each side feels like the victim of the other, and each reacts defensively, often with anger or violence. In this cycle, responsibility becomes blurred because both sides feel justified in their actions and both see the other as the aggressor.

If we apply this to antisemitism, it is important to be clear: hatred of Jews has a very long history that existed long before the State of Israel. It cannot be explained away as a response to Jewish behaviour. Antisemitism is a prejudice, a projection, and a form of hatred that Jews have endured across centuries and continents. To blame Jews for antisemitism would repeat the old logic of the oppressor, saying the victim somehow provokes their own persecution.

At the same time, Benjamin's framework helps us look at the complexity inside the Jewish community itself. When Jews criticize Israel, this is not necessarily antisemitism. It can be an act of recognition: the attempt to hold Israel accountable while affirming shared values of justice and humanity. Calling this *antisemitic* erases the difference between hatred of Jews and legitimate political or moral critique.

So the answer is twofold: Jews are not to blame for antisemitism; it is hatred projected onto them. But Jews, like all people, can and do criticize their own institutions and governments. Far from being antisemitic, such criticism can reflect Benjamin's hope that we move beyond blame and domination towards recognition, accountability, and coexistence.

As Jewish collective life has been mainly in the diaspora over the two millennia, I would suggest that the idea of the existence of an independent Jewish state is a fact that some Jewish and non-Jewish communities and individuals find hard to accept. The internalized state of diaspora, or exile from the biblical Promised Land, has become an object in individual and communal Jewish life and in the non-Jewish world.

The idea of the Jew in Exile has been very evocative as an inspiration for many Jewish thoughts throughout the ages, starting with the prophets (Isaiah,

Jeremiah, Ezekiel), moving through Maimonides and in modern times thinkers like the Jewish French-Egyptian philosopher Edmond Jabès (1912–1991), who even went so far as to claim the true homeland of the Jews is in the Hebrew language and not in any physical territory.

Jews being critical of aspects of Jewish life doesn't mean they hate themselves or their heritage. Instead, it shows they can thoughtfully examine their traditions and make informed choices about what they want to embrace, change, or leave behind.

Actually, debate and reinterpretation are fundamental to Jewish intellectual tradition. Jewish scholars have always devoted themselves to studying and restudying sacred texts, trying to understand deeper meanings in what they see as complex expressions of the divine. This ongoing process of hermeneutics, discussing, and reinterpreting is not only accepted but celebrated as a core part of Jewish thought.

In his 1939 *Moses and Monotheism*, the last essay he wrote, Freud made the claim that Judaism's strict monotheism and emphasis on ethical law provoke both admiration and resentment, leading to antisemitic attitudes. He asked what the role was that the Jewish adherence to their own way of life and set of beliefs had to play in the antisemitic drama?

Central to traditional Jewish identity is the concept that the Jews are the chosen people. Jehovah chose the Jewish people to deliver his teachings to humanity. This is a central tenet in Jewish thought, allocating the Jewish people a special, perhaps superior, place amongst other people.

Without expanding the argument too much or dealing with it in theological terms, I suggest that such a claim, the singularity and superiority of an ethnic group, can evoke a range of reactions. From a psychoanalytical point of view, if a single individual was to make such a claim that he himself is morally superior, that he also was chosen to deliver God's words to humanity, he would be thought to be either suffering from a *narcissistic personality disorder* or to be delusional.

It must be acknowledged that the two other monotheistic religions, Christianity and Islam, make similar claims. Christianity sees Jesus Christ as the incarnation of God, while Islam views Muhammad as the true prophet. When coupled with political weakness, the followers of these religions have also suffered mass persecution, as is evident in the recent persecution of Muslims in China.

The persecution of Muslims in China, particularly the Uyghur ethnic minority in the Xinjiang region, remains one of the most alarming human rights issues globally. This systemic repression encompasses cultural, religious, and personal freedoms, enforced under the guise of counterterrorism and national unity policies. There are of course many other examples whereby racial, ethnic, and religious minorities suffer from persistent persecution due to their adherence in their individual and collective identity. The idea of being chosen or singular is indeed an individual and group trait which will arouse hostility from others. Coupled with political vulnerability, it may lead to disastrous consequences. It is not within the scope of this chapter to determine whether the Jews have suffered more than other minorities, but they have certainly paid their share.

The claim that Jewish insistence on their singularity is a justified cause for antisemitism needs to be treated with great care. To begin with, antisemitism is never justified. Hatred of Jews has existed in many times and places, regardless of what Jews did or how they lived. It is a prejudice, a projection, and a way for societies to explain their problems by blaming an other.

That said, we can try to unpack the tension around Jewish singularity. Jews have often held on tightly to a sense of being unique, whether through religion, culture, history, or survival after persecution. For many Jews, this sense of uniqueness is not about superiority but about identity and continuity. After centuries of exile, pogroms, and especially the Holocaust, holding onto singularity became a way to preserve dignity and survival.

From the outside, however, this insistence has sometimes been misunderstood. Some people perceive Jewish singularity as separateness or exclusion. When mixed with resentment, ignorance, or conspiracy theories, this perception can fuel hostility. But here we need to be precise: the hostility does not come from Jewish singularity itself; it comes from how others project their fears and frustrations onto Jews.

Jessica Benjamin's framework is again useful here. The problem arises when groups get stuck in a *doer/done-to* cycle, unable to recognize each other as full human beings. Antisemitism locks Jews into the role of the *other* who is either too powerful or too different. Breaking that cycle means moving towards recognition: seeing Jewish singularity not as a threat but as one form of human difference among many.

So the plain answer is: Jewish singularity is not the cause of antisemitism. The cause lies in prejudice and projection. The challenge is how to honour uniqueness without it being turned against Jews.

The Jew as the Other

The tendency to negate the Jew as the *other* in such clear and one-dimensional terms indicates, in Kleinian terms, a regression to *the paranoid-schizoid position.*

The paranoid-schizoid position is a developmental stage which infants are supposed to go through during the first year of their lives. It culminates in the integration of the seemingly opposing forces of *love and aggression.* Once integrated, the individual reaches *the depressive* position, whereby they are able to maintain an ambivalence, realizing that nobody and nothing is perfect.

This is achieved successfully by most people, but even when that occurs, the danger of regressing back to the paranoid-schizoid position remains throughout life. At times of threat, internally or externally, most individuals would find themselves back in that position temporarily, as a means of defending themselves from being taken over by a sense of helplessness. Once the danger is over, most individuals would return to the depressive position, where they are able to uphold an ambivalent and rational attitude towards life.

Traditionally, the antisemite, at least within the Christian tradition, has held Jews responsible for betraying Jesus Christ and causing his crucifixion. I suggest that what Christians could not tolerate was not only the crucifixion itself but the unbearable feelings stirred by imagining such an injury done to Christ. To rid themselves of this inner torment, they projected it outward. By attributing the pain to the Jews, they could see themselves as righteous and the Jews as evil.

When someone imagines something terrible, it is still their own mind doing the imagining. The thought belongs to them; they are the agent of it. No one forces such thoughts upon them. Yet, to avoid taking responsibility for these dark imaginings, people may project them onto others.

In this case, Jews came to be seen as responsible for causing the crisis and as benefitting from it. Such an accusation reflects *paranoid anxiety*: a state in which a person feels persecuted by an external *bad object* that they believe threatens their well-being. This anxiety arises when someone cannot clearly distinguish between their own inner fears and external reality. To manage such anxiety, people fall back on primitive defences like denial, idealization, or fantasies of omnipotent control.

In this mental state, the Jew is not experienced as a whole person but as *a part-object*, a fragment embodying danger and malice. Once reduced to this status, Jews could be treated inhumanely, as if destroying them would eliminate the imagined threat. This mechanism helps explain how *civilised* people in Europe, such as Germans and their neighbours, could commit atrocities against Jews during World War II despite having lived in seemingly ordinary relationships with them before the war.

This emotional configuration echoes Freud's account of how children manage forbidden incestuous desires. In both early development and puberty, the child naturally experiences deep attachment to the mother, the first source of sensory pleasure. As Freud argued in *Three Essays on the Theory of Sexuality*, these early bodily experiences later inform sexual development. Inevitably, fantasies of union with the mother arise. The oedipal prohibition transforms these fantasies: direct incest is forbidden, but desire is displaced onto other objects. If this inhibitory system fails, however, we may encounter perversion or abuse, where intolerable fantasies are acted out rather than managed symbolically. In healthier development, the intolerable fantasy is redirected or transformed.

In the same way, the antisemite disowns the unbearable fantasy of Christ's crucifixion. Rather than acknowledging it as part of himself, he projects it onto Jews, who are then hated as carriers of what he cannot accept in his own mind. By attempting to annihilate Jews, he is in fact trying to annihilate the intolerable part of himself.

Of course, the crucifixion fantasy is not the only projection fuelling antisemitism. It is simply one example of how such mechanisms can work. Once established in individuals, these projections and anxieties become available for political leaders and movements to exploit for their own purposes, turning inner emotional conflicts into destructive social realities.

I will conclude this discussion by suggesting that the recent upsurge of antisemitic attacks after the 7th October murderous Hamas assault is linked, amongst other factors, to the fact that Israel has acted in ways which are not dissimilar to what other modern states would have done. It has responded with tremendous force to having been attacked and having its citizens held in captivity for more than twenty months (at the time when this chapter was written) without an end to captivity in sight. It has shown again that as a society it is strong, despite internal disputes, and has employed considerable military force against its enemies.

This has prompted severe international condemnation, which is at times seen as thinly disguised antisemitism. From a psychoanalytical point of view, I suggest that such criticism, even if partially justified, reveals a deeply ingrained view of Jews as weak victims, deserving to be persecuted as they claim to be God's chosen people and therefore needing to rely only upon their moral ethics and not seek actual political power. In psychoanalytic terms, the criticism towards Israel for defending its borders and citizens, something all states would do, is in fact *reaction formation*.

Jews have claimed themselves to be morally superior while being a minority. Once they established themselves as a majority in the state of Israel, it was soon discovered that their individual and collective behaviour is no different than any other community or state. Thus, the Jewish claim to be superior and singular has been refuted and aroused unconscious outrage. It seems as if there was indeed a tacit agreement that the Jews and Judaism were somehow singular, perhaps due to them being around longer than any other minority, at least in the monotheistic world, and so discovering that they are not so singular or even more moral than others has evoked a sense of disappointment and betrayal, which is being vented out through the recent antisemitic outrage.

In a sense, it is as if the world has been awakened to the fact that the Jews are no different to others and will react in ways which are very similar to other communities and nation when feeling threatened. Therefore, the Jewish claim to be singular has acted as a double-edged sword: on the one hand it has provided a sense of uniqueness but on the other it has created false expectations, leading to a severe universal sense of disappointment. Now, the time is perhaps ripe for Jews and non-Jews alike to acknowledge that Jews have no superiority or singularity and are to be treated the same as other communities and nations, for better and for worse.

Where Do We Go from Here?

> *The voice of the intellect is a soft one, but it does not rest until it has gained a hearing. Ultimately, after endless rebuffs, it succeeds. This is one of the few points in which one may be optimistic about the future of mankind.*
>
> (Freud, 1933, p. 163)

To end a chapter, and even more so an entire book, with a single statement is always difficult. Any attempt will fall short of the complexity of our times. And yet, in an age marked by peril, rupture, and uncertainty whether in the Middle East or across the globe, there remains a truth worth holding on to: hope depends upon our willingness to preserve a sense of rational and creative agency. *To surrender to despair is to abandon what makes us human.* Instead, we are called to act with creativity and courage, to extend towards one another the attentive, non-judgemental compassion and the firm respect that psychoanalysis has taught us to value. In this lies the possibility of repair, both personal and collective.

About the Author

Rony Alfandary, Ph.D. is a clinical social worker and senior lecturer at the School of Social Work at the University of Haifa. He served as Director of the Post-Graduate Programme in Psychoanalytic Psychotherapy at Bar-Ilan University until 2022.

Rony graduated from Trent Polytechnic, Nottingham, England, in 1986 with a BA (Honours) in Photography. He earned his MA (CCETSW) in Social Work at Nottingham University in 1992 and completed a three-year postgraduate programme in psychoanalytic psychotherapy at the Bar-Ilan University in 1998. He received his Ph.D. from the Program for Hermeneutics and Cultural Studies at the Bar-Ilan University in 2012.

His research interests are multidisciplinary, encompassing psychoanalytic social work, photography, hermeneutics, the relationships between language, creativity, and the sense of self and belonging, as well as the impact of the Holocaust on second and third generations.

Rony represents the Israeli Association of Psychoanalytic Psychotherapy (IAPP) as a board member of the World Council of Psychotherapy (WCP) and the European Federation of Psychoanalytic Psychotherapy (EFPP). He is also a founding member of the Israeli voluntary organization *The Road to Recovery*, which helps hundreds of Palestinian children from the West Bank and Gaza access medical care in Israeli hospitals, serving in various capacities including Chairman of the Board in 2022–2023.

As well as practising psychoanalytic psychotherapy, he engages in still photography and film-making, with a diverse portfolio spanning theatre, disability, street photography, and documentary work. He has published twelve books and numerous articles, including two volumes of poetry (2004 and 2023) and two novels (2000 and 2022).

More can be seen on his website www.ronyalfandary.com

DOI: 10.4324/9781003683162-12

Selected Academic and Clinical Publications

2013

Alfandary, R. (2013). Dreaming in Alexandria [In Hebrew]. Ma'arg, 4, 69–98.

2014

Alfandary, R. (2014). An exile in the room: A clinical illustration and a literary footnote. Psychoanalytic Social Work, 22(1), 23–38.

2015

Alfandary, R. (2015). An instance of emotional absence of a father traumatized by war. American Journal of Psychotherapy, 69(1), 1–17.

2016

Alfandary, R. (2016). Transference-love and institutional involvement in a case of psychotherapy supervision. Psychoanalytic Social Work, 23(1), 60–71.

Alfandary, R. (2016). Galut ve Hitgalut: A psychoanalytical study of Lawrence Durrell's The Alexandria Quartet [In Hebrew]. Carmel Publishers.

Alfandary, R. (2016). To write or not to write – is that the question? [In Hebrew]. Ma'arg, 7, 1–18.

2018

Alfandary, R. (Ed.). (2018). Seeking psychic space: Fundamentals of psychodynamic social work (Vol. 1) [In Hebrew]. Carmel Publishers.

2019

Alfandary, R. (2019). Exile and return: A psychoanalytical study of Lawrence Durrell's The Alexandria Quartet. Routledge.

Alfandary, R. (2019). The invisible wound: A study of the emotional abuse of children. Lambert Academic Publishing.

2020

Alfandary, R. (2020). Concerning Israeli psyche – The uncanny dimension of COVID-19 [In Hebrew]. Society and Welfare, M2–3, 233–236.

Alfandary, R. (2020). Leaving home and adolescence in Lawrence Durrell's Pied Piper of Lovers: A psychoanalytic reading. In R. Pine & V. Konidari (Eds.), Islands of the mind: Psychology, literature and biodiversity (pp. 176–193). Cambridge Scholars Publishing.

Alfandary, R. (2020). To be a refugee: Testimony of a Jewish Bulgarian family, 1941–1948. In S. Steinberg & A. Grenville (Eds.), Refugees from Nazi-occupied Europe in British Overseas Territories (pp. 119–140). Brill Rodopi.

Alfandary, R. (2020). Exile and return in Julio Cortázar's work [In Hebrew]. In D. Lemberger (Ed.), The soul beetle (pp. 217–246). Resling Books.

Alfandary, R. (2020). The lone photograph [In Hebrew]. In H. Erel-Brodsky (Ed.), Criss-cross: Psychoanalysis, art and culture (pp. 85–98). Resling Books.

Alfandary, R. (2020). Writing about COVID. In J. Baumel-Schwartz (Ed.), Creating under COVID. Bar-Ilan University Publishers.

2021

Alfandary, R. (2021). Stories from boxes. The Journal of Greek Holocaust Survivors [In Hebrew], 36, 40–41.

Alfandary, R. (2021). Post-memory, psychoanalysis and Holocaust ghosts: The Salonica Cohen family and trauma across generations. C.20 – An International Journal, December 2021. The Durrell Library of Corfu.

2022

Alfandary, R. (2022). Post-memory, psychoanalysis and Holocaust ghosts. Routledge.

2023

Alfandary, R., & Baumel-Schwartz, J. (2023). Psychoanalytic and cultural aspects of trauma and the Holocaust. Routledge.

2024

Alfandary, R. (Ed.). (2024). Seeking psychic space: Fundamentals of psychodynamic social work (Vol. 2) [In Hebrew]. Carmel Publishers.

2025

Alfandary, R. (2025). Psychoanalysis and antisemitism. Vestigia, 4(2), 23–31.

Further Reading

Akhtar, S. (2013). *Psychoanalytic listening: Methods, limits and innovations.* Karnac.

Alvarez, A. (1992). *Live company: Psychoanalytic psychotherapy with autistic, borderline, deprived and abused children.* Routledge.

Anastasopoulos, D., & Tsiantis, J. (1999). Supervision of individual psychoanalytic psychotherapy in institutions: The setting, the dynamics and the learning process. *Psychoanalytic Psychotherapy*, 13(2), 167–183.

Appelfeld, A. (2004). *The story of a life* (A. Halter, Trans.). Schocken Books.

Arendt, H. (1958). *The human condition*. University of Chicago Press.

Aron, L. (2006). Analytic impasse and the third: Clinical implications of intersubjective theory. *International Journal of Psychoanalysis*, 87(2), 349–368.

Austin, J. L. (1975). *How to do things with words.* Oxford University Press.

Bakhtin, M. (1965). *Rabelais and his world.* MIT Press.

Barthes, R. (1972). *Mythologies.* Paladin Books.

Basch, M. F. (1980). *Doing psychotherapy.* Basic Books.

Benjamin, J. (2018). *Beyond doer and done to: Recognition theory, intersubjectivity and the third.* Routledge.

Berman, E. (1993). Introduction. In E. Berman (Ed.), *Essential papers on literature and psychoanalysis* (pp. 1–18). New York University Press.

Bernstein, S. B. (2008). Writing, rewriting, and working-through. *Psychoanalytic Inquiry*, 28(3), 450–464.

Bertin, C. (1983). *Marie Bonaparte: A life.* Quartet Books.

Bhabha, H. (1992). The world and the home. *Social Text*, 31/32, 141–152.

Bion, W. R. (1959). Attacks on linking. *International Journal of Psycho-Analysis*, 40, 308–315.

Blos, P. (1962). *On adolescence: A psychoanalytic interpretation*. Free Press.

Bollas, C. (1989). *Forces of destiny.* Free Association Books.

Bollas, C. (1994). Aspects of the erotic transference. *Psychoanalytic Inquiry*, 14(4), 572–590.

Bollas, C. (1995). The structure of evil. In *Cracking up* (pp. 180–220). Routledge.

Bolognini, S. (1994). Transference: Erotised, erotic, loving, affectionate. *International Journal of Psycho-Analysis*, 75, 73–86.

Bos, E. (2019). Why are arts-based interventions useful in social work practice? In E. Huss & E. Bos (Eds.), *Arts in social work practice* (pp. 11–17). Routledge.

Botèro, H. (2012). When father is not there: The absence of the father as a generating factor of violence. *International Journal of Applied Psychoanalytic Studies*, 9(2), 109–133.

Bowker, G. (1997). *Through the dark labyrinth: A biography of Lawrence Durrell*. St. Martin's Press.

Bowlby, J. (1969). *Attachment* (Vol. 1 of Attachment and loss). Basic Books.

Bowlby, J. (1973). *Separation: Anxiety and anger* (Vol. 2 of Attachment and loss). Basic Books.

Bowlby, J. (1980). *Loss: Sadness and depression* (Vol. 3 of Attachment and loss). Basic Books.

Breuer, J., & Freud, S. (1895). *Studies on hysteria* (J. Strachey, Trans. & Ed.). In J. Strachey (Ed. & Trans.), The standard edition of the complete psychological works of Sigmund Freud (Vol. 2, pp. 1–305). Hogarth Press.

Caligor, L., Bromberg, P., & Meltzer, J. (1984). *Clinical perspectives on the supervision of psychoanalysis and psychotherapy*. Plenum Press.

Camus, A. (1948). *The plague*. Vintage International.

Casement, P. (1985). *On learning from the patient*. Routledge.

Casement, P. (1990). *Further learning from the patient: The analytic space and process*. Routledge.

Collins, S. (2011). On authenticity: The question of truth in construction and autobiography. *International Journal of Psychoanalysis*, 92(6), 1391–1409.

Cortázar, J. (1979). *All fires the fire*. Marion Boyars.

Cortázar, J. (2005). *Diary of Andrés Fava*. Archipelago Books.

Cortázar, J. (2013). *Literature class*. New Directions.

Cuijpers, P., Karyotaki, E., Ebert, D. D., … & Furukawa, T. A. (2024). Absolute and relative outcomes of psychotherapies for eight mental disorders: A systematic review and meta-analysis. *World Psychiatry*, 23(1), 65–81.

Davies, J. M., & Frawley, M. G. (1994). *Treating the adult survivor of childhood sexual abuse* (Vol. 1). Basic Books.

Denford, J. (1981). Going away. *International Review of Psychoanalysis*, 8, 325–332.

Dick, G. L. (2011). The changing role of fatherhood: The father as a provider of self-object functions. *Psychoanalytic Social Work*, 18(1), 107–125.

Doehrman, M. (1976). Parallel processes in supervision and psychotherapy. *Bulletin of the Menninger Clinic*, 40(2), 9–110.

Durrell, L. (1957). *Justine*. Faber & Faber.

Durrell, L. (1958a). *Balthazar*. Faber & Faber.

Durrell, L. (1958b). *Mountolive*. Faber & Faber.

Durrell, L. (1960). *Clea*. Faber & Faber.

Durrell, L. ([1935] 2008). *Pied piper of lovers*. ELS Editions.

Durrell, S. (1991). Journals and letters. In *The family: They fuck you up* (pp. 55–92). Granta.

Eigan, M. (2018). *Toxic nourishment*. Routledge.

Felman, S. (1977). *Literature and psychoanalysis*. Johns Hopkins University Press.

Felman, S. (2003). *Writing and madness*. Stanford University Press.

Felman, S., & Laub, D. (1992). *Testimony: Crises of witnessing in literature, psychoanalysis, and history*. Routledge.

Fonagy, P., & Allison, E. (2014). The role of mentalizing and epistemic trust in the therapeutic relationship. *Psychotherapy*, 51(3), 372–380.

Foucault, M. (1970). *The order of things.* Pantheon Books.
Foucault, M. (1997). What is critique? In *The politics of truth* (pp. 41–82). Semiotext(e).
Fowler, H. W., & Fowler, F. G. (1982). *The concise Oxford dictionary.* Clarendon Press.
Frankl, V. E. (1959). *Man's search for meaning.* Beacon Press.
Freud, E. L. (Ed.). (1960). *The letters of Sigmund Freud* (T. & J. Stern, Trans.). Basic Books.
Freud, M. (1958). *Sigmund Freud: Man and father.* Vanguard Press.
Freud, S. (1896). *Further remarks on the neuro-psychoses of defence.* In J. Strachey (Ed. & Trans.), The standard edition of the complete psychological works of Sigmund Freud (Vol. 3, pp. 159–174). Hogarth Press.
Freud, S. (1899). *Screen memories* (J. Strachey, Trans.). In J. Strachey (Ed. & Trans.), The standard edition of the complete psychological works of Sigmund Freud (Vol. 23, pp. 299–322). Hogarth Press.
Freud, S. (1900). *The interpretation of dreams.* In J. Strachey (Ed. & Trans.), The standard edition of the complete psychological works of Sigmund Freud (Vols. 4–5). Hogarth Press.
Freud, S. (1905). *Three essays on the theory of sexuality.* In J. Strachey (Ed. & Trans.), The standard edition of the complete psychological works of Sigmund Freud (Vol. 7, pp. 123–245). Hogarth Press.
Freud, S. (1908). *Creative writers and day-dreaming.* In J. Strachey (Ed. & Trans.), The standard edition of the complete psychological works of Sigmund Freud (Vol. 9, pp. 143–153). Hogarth Press.
Freud, S. (1912). *Recommendations to physicians practising psycho-analysis.* In J. Strachey (Ed. & Trans.), The standard edition of the complete psychological works of Sigmund Freud (Vol. 12, pp. 109–120). Hogarth Press.
Freud, S. (1913). *On beginning the treatment (Further recommendations on the technique of psycho-analysis I).* In J. Strachey (Ed. & Trans.), The standard edition of the complete psychological works of Sigmund Freud (Vol. 12, pp. 121–144). Hogarth Press.
Freud, S. (1914). *Some reflections on schoolboy psychology.* In J. Strachey (Ed. & Trans.), The standard edition of the complete psychological works of Sigmund Freud (Vol. 13, pp. 307–326). Hogarth Press.
Freud, S. (1915a). *Observations on transference-love.* In J. Strachey (Ed. & Trans.), The standard edition of the complete psychological works of Sigmund Freud (Vol. 12, pp. 159–171). Hogarth Press.
Freud, S. (1915b). *Repression.* In J. Strachey (Ed. & Trans.), The standard edition of the complete psychological works of Sigmund Freud (Vol. 14, pp. 141–159). Hogarth Press.
Freud, S. (1915c). *The unconscious.* In J. Strachey (Ed. & Trans.), The standard edition of the complete psychological works of Sigmund Freud (Vol. 14, pp. 159–216). Hogarth Press.
Freud, S. (1917). *Mourning and melancholia.* In J. Strachey (Ed. & Trans.), The standard edition of the complete psychological works of Sigmund Freud (Vol. 14, pp. 237–258). Hogarth Press.
Freud, S. (1919). *The uncanny* (J. Strachey, Trans.). In J. Strachey (Ed. & Trans.), The standard edition of the complete psychological works of Sigmund Freud (Vol. 17, pp. 217–256). Hogarth Press.
Freud, S. (1920). *Beyond the pleasure principle* (J. Strachey, Trans.). In J. Strachey (Ed. & Trans.), The standard edition of the complete psychological works of Sigmund Freud (Vol. 18, pp. 7–64). Hogarth Press.

Freud, S. (1927). *The future of an illusion.* In J. Strachey (Ed. & Trans.), The standard edition of the complete psychological works of Sigmund Freud (Vol. 21, pp. 21–56). Hogarth Press.

Freud, S. (1930). *Civilization and its discontents.* In J. Strachey (Ed. & Trans.), The standard edition of the complete psychological works of Sigmund Freud (Vol. 21, pp. 57–146). Hogarth Press.

Freud, S. (1933). *New introductory lectures on psycho-analysis* (J. Strachey, Trans.). In J. Strachey (Ed. & Trans.), The standard edition of the complete psychological works of Sigmund Freud (Vols. 22–23). Hogarth Press.

Freud, S. (1937). *Analysis terminable and interminable* (J. Strachey, Trans.). In J. Strachey (Ed. & Trans.), The standard edition of the complete psychological works of Sigmund Freud (Vol. 23, pp. 209–254). Hogarth Press.

Freud, S. (1939). *Moses and monotheism.* In J. Strachey (Ed. & Trans.), The standard edition of the complete psychological works of Sigmund Freud (Vol. 23, pp. 1–137). Hogarth Press.

Freud, S. (1954). *The origins of psychoanalysis: Letters to Wilhelm Fliess, drafts and notes: 1887–1902* (M. Bonaparte, A. Freud, & E. Kris, Eds.; E. Mosbacher & J. Strachey, Trans.). Basic Books.

Freud, S. (1960). *Letters of Sigmund Freud.* McGraw-Hill.

Fromm-Reichmann, F. (1950). *Principles of intensive psychotherapy.* University of Chicago Press.

Frosh, S. (2013). *Hauntings: Psychoanalysis and ghostly transmissions.* Palgrave Macmillan.

Gabbard, G. O. (2000). Disguise or consent: Problems and recommendations concerning the publication and presentation of clinical material. *International Journal of Psycho-Analysis,* 81(5), 1071–1086.

Gabbard, G. (2006). Sexual and nonsexual boundary violation in psychoanalysis and psychotherapy. In S. Akhtar (Ed.), *Interpersonal boundaries: Variations and violations* (pp. 39–48). Jason Aronson.

Gadamer, H.-G. (2004). *Truth and interpretation.* Continuum.

Gay, P. (1989). *Freud: A life for our times.* Papermac.

Gay, P. (1990). *Reading Freud.* Yale University Press.

Goldberg, A. (1997). Writing case histories. *International Journal of Psycho-Analysis,* 78(3), 435–438.

Goldberg, F. (1990). Contemporary issues and approaches to psychoanalytic supervision. In R. Lane (Ed.), *Psychoanalytic approaches to supervision.* Brunner.

Goldberg, P. (1989). Actively seeking the holding environment: Conscious and unconscious elements in the building of a therapeutic framework. *Contemporary Psychoanalysis,* 25(4), 448–453.

Govrin, A. (2015). *Conservative and radical perspectives on psychoanalytic knowledge: The fascinated and the disenchanted.* Routledge.

Green, A. (1986). *On private madness* (A. Weller, Trans.). International Universities Press. (Original work published 1980)

Green, A. (1998). The primordial mind and the work of the negative. *International Journal of Psychoanalysis,* 79(4), 649–667.

Greenberg, J. R., & Mitchell, S. A. (1983). *Object relations in psychoanalytic theory.* Harvard University Press.

Grinberg, L., & Grinberg, R. (1989). *Psychoanalytic perspectives on migration and exile*. Yale University Press.
Guntrip, H. (1974). *Schizoid phenomena, object-relations and the self*. Hogarth Press.
Hanly, C. (2009). On truth and clinical psychoanalysis. *International Journal of Psycho-Analysis*, 90(2), 363–373.
Heidegger, M. (1959). *Discourse on thinking* (J. M. Anderson & E. H. Freund, Trans.). Harper & Row.
Howard, S. (2007). Models of supervision. In A. Petts & B. Shapely (Eds.), *On supervision: Psychoanalytic and Jungian perspectives*. Karnac Books.
Kalmanowitz, D., Huss, E., & Bos, E. (2023). Social action art therapy: An Israeli context. In E. Huss & E. Bos (Eds.), *Using art for social transformation* (pp. 19–32). Routledge.
Kantrowitz, J. L. (2004). Writing about patients: Ways of protecting confidentiality and analysts' conflicts over choice of method. *Journal of the American Psychoanalytic Association*, 52(1), 69–99.
Kanzer, M. (1950). The Oedipus trilogy. *Psychoanalytic Quarterly*, 19(4), 561–572.
Karon, B. (1990). Psychoanalysis, psychoanalytic therapy and the process of supervision. In R. Lane (Ed.), *Psychoanalytic approaches to supervision*. Brunner.
Kernberg, O. (1970). A psychoanalytic classification of character pathology. *Journal of the American Psychoanalytic Association*, 18(4), 800–822.
Klein, M. (1986). *The selected Melanie Klein* (J. Mitchell, Ed.). Free Press.
Kohut, H. (1977). *The restoration of the self*. University of Chicago Press.
Kristeva, J. (1991). *Strangers to ourselves*. Columbia University Press.
Laplanche, J., & Pontalis, J.-B. (1973). *The language of psychoanalysis*. Karnac Books.
Laub, D., & Felman, S. (1992). *Testimony*. Routledge.
Leichsenring, F., Steinert, C., Hoyer, J., Rabung, S., & Salanti, G. (2022). The efficacy of psychotherapies and pharmacotherapies for mental disorders in adults: An umbrella review and meta-analytic evaluation of recent meta-analyses. *World Psychiatry*, 21(1), 133–145.
Lessing, T. (2021). *Jewish self-hate* (P. C. Applebaum, Trans.). Berghahn Books.
Levy, R. S. (Ed.). (2005). *Antisemitism: A historical encyclopaedia of prejudice and persecution* (Vols. 1–2). ABC-CLIO.
Lloyd-Owen, D. (1997). From action to thought: Supervising mental health workers with forensic patients. In B. Martindale, M. Morner, M. E. C. Rodriguez, & J. P. Vidit (Eds.), *Supervision and its vicissitudes*. Karnac Books.
Luber, M. P. (1991). Patient's transference to the analyst's supervisor: Effect of the setting on the analytic process. *Journal of the American Psychoanalytic Association*, 39(3), 705–725.
Lugar, S. (2013). Father figure: On dangerous daddies and cross-generational desire. *Studies in Gender and Sexuality*, 14(2), 153–157.
MacNiven, I. S. (1998). *Lawrence Durrell: A biography*. Faber & Faber.
Marshall, E. (1986). Causal explanation in science and in psychoanalysis – Implications for writing a case study. *Psychoanalytic Study of the Child*, 41, 89–127.
Michels, R. (2000). The case history. *Journal of the American Psychoanalytic Association*, 48(2), 355–375.
Mills, J. M. (2011). Deconstructing Hermes: A critique of the hermeneutic turn in psychoanalysis. *American Journal of Psychoanalysis*, 71(3), 238–245.
Nägele, R. (1978). *Reading after Freud*. Columbia University Press.

Nin, A. (1967). *The journals of Anaïs Nin: Vol. 6, 1955–1966*. Quartet Books.
Ogden, B. H., & Ogden, T. H. (2013). *The analyst's ear and the critic's eye: Rethinking psychoanalysis and literature*. Routledge.
Ogden, T. H. (1986). *The matrix of the mind*. Jason Aronson.
Ogden, T. H. (1997). Some thoughts on the use of language in psychoanalysis. *Psychoanalytic Dialogues*, 7(1), 1–21.
Ogden, T. H. (2002). *The primitive edge of experience*. Jason Aronson.
Ogden, T. H. (2004). The analytic third: Implications for psychoanalytic theory and technique. *Psychoanalytic Quarterly*, 73(2), 167–195.
Parsons, M. (2000). *The dove that returns, the dove that vanishes*. Routledge.
Perelberg, R. J. (2009). Murdered father; dead father: Revisiting the Oedipus complex. *The International Journal of Psychoanalysis*, 90(4), 713–732.
Philips, A. (2002). *Promises, promises: Essays on literature and psychoanalysis*. Basic Books.
Pine, R. (2005). *Lawrence Durrell: The mindscape* (2nd ed.). Durrell School of Corfu.
Poland, W. S. (2009). Problems of collegial learning in psychoanalysis: Narcissism and curiosity. *International Journal of Psycho-Analysis*, 90(3), 249–262.
Quinodoz, J.-M. (2005). *Reading Freud*. Routledge.
Ricoeur, P. (1970). *Freud and philosophy: An essay on interpretation* (D. Savage, Trans.). Yale University Press.
Rogers, C. R. (1961). *On becoming a person: A therapist's view of psychotherapy*. Houghton Mifflin.
Roth, M. (2020). *A psychoanalytic perspective on reading literature: Reading the reader* (D. Gillon, Trans.). Routledge.
Sagi, A. (2002). *Albert Camus and the philosophy of the absurd*. Editions Rodopi.
Sagi, A. (2015). *Living with the other: The ethic of inner retreat*. Springer.
Sagi, A. (2017). *Reflections on identity: The Jewish case*. Academic Studies Press.
Sandler, J., Dare, C., & Holder, A. (1992). *The patient and the analyst: The basis of the psychoanalytic process*. Karnac Books.
Sartre, J.-P. (1980). *Anti-Semite and Jew* (G. J. Becker, Trans.). Schocken Books.
Schafer, R. (1997). Vicissitudes of remembering in the countertransference: Fervent, failure, colonization and remembering otherwise. *International Journal of Psychoanalysis*, 78(5), 1151–1163.
Searles, H. (1955). The informational value of the supervisor's emotional experiences. *Psychiatry*, 18(2), 135–146.
Searles, H. F. (1960). *The non-human environment*. International Universities Press.
Searles, H. F. (1963). Transference psychosis in the psychotherapy of chronic schizophrenia. *International Journal of Psycho-Analysis*, 44(2), 249–281.
Sher, M. (2003). Ethical issues for psychotherapists working in organizations. In H. Solomon & M. Twyman (Eds.), *Ethics in contemporary psychotherapy practice*. Free Association Books.
Simpson, J. (Ed.). (1995). *The Oxford book of exile*. Oxford University Press.
Solms, M. (2021). *The hidden spring: A journey to the source of consciousness*. W. W. Norton & Company.
Spence, D. P. (2003). Listening for rhetorical truth. *Psychoanalytic Quarterly*, 83(4), 875–903.
Spence, D. P. (2007). Perils and pitfalls of memory-based reporting: How case histories can become more evidence-based. *Psychoanalytic Inquiry*, 27(5), 602–616.

Spero, M. H. (2010). The transformations in the "mental apparatus of dreaming" as depicted in the biblical story of Joseph (Genesis 40–43). In *Contemporary psychoanalysis and Judaism* (pp. 186–235). Academic Studies Press.
Spero, M. H. (2026). What time does the analytic hour begin? Introducing the "intrapsychic temporal threshold representation". *American Journal of Psychoanalysis*, 86(1). [In process].
Steiner, G. (1978). A remark on language and psychoanalysis. In *On difficulty and other essays* (pp. 48–61). Oxford University Press.
Steiner, R. (1989). It is a new kind of diaspora. *International Review of Psycho-Analysis*, 16(1), 35–78.
Stern, D. N. (1985). *The interpersonal world of the infant*. Basic Books.
Stoller, R. (1988). Patients' responses to their own case reports. *Journal of the American Psychoanalytic Association*, 36(2), 371–391.
Szajnberg, N. M. (1992). Psychoanalysis as an extension of the autobiographical genre: Poetry and truth, fiction and reality. *International Review of Psycho-Analysis*, 9(4), 375–387.
Szecsody, I. (1990). Supervision: A didactic or mutative situation. *Psychoanalytic Psychotherapy*, 4(3), 245–261.
Thomas, D. M. (1981). *The white hotel*. Penguin Books.
Tuckett, D. (2000). Reporting clinical events in the journal: Towards the construction of a special case. *International Journal of Psycho-Analysis*, 81(5), 1065–1069.
Turner, V. (1969). *The ritual process: Structure and anti-structure*. Aldine Transaction.
Wallerstein, R. (1981). *Becoming a psychoanalyst: A study of psychoanalytic supervision*. International Universities Press.
Winnicott, D. W. (1950). Aggression in relation to emotional development. In D. W. Winnicott, *The maturational processes and the facilitating environment* (pp. 214–215). International Universities Press.
Winnicott, D. W. (1958). Primitive emotional development. In *Through paediatrics to Psycho-Analysis* (pp. 145–156). Tavistock Publications.
Winnicott, D. W. (1958). *Through paediatrics to psychoanalysis*. Karnac Books.
Winnicott, D. W. (1960). The theory of the parent–infant relationship. In D. W. Winnicott, *The maturational processes and the facilitating environment: Studies in the theory of emotional development* (pp. 37–55). Karnac Books.
Winnicott, D. W. (1962a). Ego integration in child development. In D. W. Winnicott, *The maturational processes and the facilitating environment* (pp. 56–63). International Universities Press.
Winnicott, D. W. (1962b). On the use of an object. In *Psychoanalytic explorations*. Karnac Books.
Winnicott, D. W. (1971). *Playing and reality*. Routledge.
Winnicott, D. W. (1986). Concept of the false self. In *Home is where we start from* (pp. 65–70). Penguin.
Wolberg, R. L. (1977). Supervision of the psychotherapeutic process. In *The technique of psychotherapy*. Grune & Stratton.
Zerubavel, N., & Wright, M. O. D. (2012). The dilemma of the wounded healer. *Psychotherapy*, 49(4), 482–491.

Index